CHALLENGES

CHALLENGES

The Norwich State Hospital Closure with Unpublished Facts and Fallout

WILFRED ZINAVAGE

LitPrime Solutions
21250 Hawthorne Blvd
Suite 500, Torrance, CA 90503
www.litprime.com
Phone: 1-800-981-9893

Published by LitPrime Solutions   01/11/2023

ISBN: 979-8-88703-130-9(sc)
ISBN: 979-8-88703-131-6(hc)
ISBN: 979-8-88703-132-3(e)

Library of Congress Control Number: 2022923701

CONTENTS

DEDICATION

This book is dedicated to the many doctors, nurses and the employees who were affected by its closure. It is also dedicated to the families of the patients and to future planners.

INTRODUCTION

Warning! Do not read this book if you are not naturally curious, enjoy history, want to learn, and meet challenges. If you're a medical professional, you will be able to understand it a little better than most.

In 1904, near the City of Norwich, Connecticut, the State of Connecticut opened a facility called Norwich Hospital for the Insane. Later, it was known as the Norwich State Hospital. Sadly, it completely closed in 1996.

In book number 3 by Bill Stanley Books in 1997, (these books are no longer in print), Mr. Stanley describes a long-ago time,

> "It was in the 1970s when, on reflection, it seems to me the world went mad. One of the do good policies was that mental patients had rights and that if they were no threat to themselves or to anyone else, they would be released. We now know that they were released into the streets of Norwich. Throughout all of the nation, the same thing was being repeated. From New York City of Los Angeles, and in any small town with a state hospital nearby, patients were

released and hospitals closed. Today, when I read the newspaper accounts, watch television, and listen to reported talk of the homeless problems, I am convinced that at least 80% of the homeless are in reality mental patients that we, as a civilized society, should be caring for."

From the time Mr. Stanley wrote this until this present date, I cannot help but wonder if some of these people didn't infiltrate our political system. For example, the City of Norwich has a mass transportation center next to a sewer plant, a rusty railroad bridge that was once a main line, and a former transportation railroadcenter now occupied by the Norwich Bulletin. Near to it is an abandoned YMCA building, "there are several other examples that local residents know about. As to the political climate in our state at the present time, it cannot help but make one wonder what the future will bring.

I present the next two statistical reports, dated June and July 1953 (author[s] unknown), which are completely uncensored or edited, as a glimpse into the past. (Note I had to add page numbers.) I believe these reports were not meant to be seen by the public and were produced only for the supervisors and administrators to read. Fortunately, they were rescued from the trash and lay dormant in an attic for decades. Note that the June report is missing pages 1 and 2, most likely from an accident. Some minor issues occurred during the reproduction, and the ink faded over time. These reports open a window for historians and medical professionals as well as the curious to glimpse what life was like in a mental health facility in the 1950s. They will also provide some insight as to how the patients were treated. Donated was a report dated November 1992 that was censored by me and other items that may be of interest.

It is ironic that the Mohegan Tribe, which once owned all the land that Norwich and surrounding towns of Sprague and Lisbon are built upon in a nine-square-mile region, later built a world-class casino, which became a city unto itself. The Mohegans repurchased the land that the state hospital once called home, and plans are underway to build a world-class theme park.

About two years ago, I found the following two reports in a box of stored documents. The more I studied them, the more I began to realize that they were reports that were made for the supervisors and administrators of the Norwich State Hospital and not meant for the public to read.

Realizing that I may run into some obstacles, I called the Connecticut State Library and told them of my find and asked them if they had such files in their library. They said no and requested that I send them these two reports.

The other concern I had is that these reports contained names of former patients and employees of the hospital. Although these reports were dated June and July 1953, nearly sixty-nine years ago, there would likely be no major concern of their release and perhaps might provide closure for some of the families included in the reports.

There are many interesting facts in these reports. Doctors, nurses, or for that matter, anyone interested in the subject of insanity may be interested. The first challenge for you, the reader, is to study them and draw your own conclusions. Remember the facts that in 1905, when the hospital was built, the challenges were different. There were no so-called miracle drugs, no cures for some sexual diseases, and the subject of post-traumatic stress disorder (PTSD) was unknown as were several other mental health maladies.

People asked me why I chose to write about the Norwich State Hospital. As I read the reports, I found them fascinating, and in them was one particular note. That note stated that in July 1953, a lobotomy was performed. Such a tiny detail!

It is my belief that that operation was performed on my uncle Anthony (ref: The Zinavage Legacy). In the history of the state hospital, I believe it was the only such operation that was performed, as at the time, it was considered experimental.

On a personal note, circa summer 1962, I took it upon myself to visit my uncle and take him out to lunch. He did not want to leave the hospital. I said to him, "Come on. I will get you a fresh cup of coffee." Again he indicated he did not want to leave the premises. His response was, "I get fresh coffee here every day." Then he said (as he removed a huge ring of keys from his pocket), "Come on. Let *me* give *you* a tour of my world."

I mentioned the keys to him, as to me, they signified a man who had access to a lot of areas. He smiled and said, "Yes, they consider me a trustee. I can get into areas that the doctors cannot, and they have come to me for access." As if to prove the point, he used his keys and said, "Let me show you where they perform water therapy." He opened the door, and I saw a twelve-by-twelve-foot room completely covered in white tiles with the center floor with a hole in it for drainage and, interestingly enough, a huge ring. I guess he read my mind as he replied, "They bring them in here naked and chain them to the ring. Then they put high-pressure hoses on them using cold water." Needless to say, I was a bit shocked, as I had never heard of such a thing. The tour continued, and I really don't remember much of it except for the following:

Still recovering from the shock, I continued to follow him as he led me through the halls to a window that was covered with heavy metal screening, and he said, "Take a look." What I saw through that window was a group of about fifteen to twenty women. Some were very beautiful. They wandered about, some aimlessly and others chatting with each other. I guess my uncle must have seen the confusion on my face, and anticipating my next question, he said, "These women are here because they loved their men too much." It took me a long time to figure that one out. They were mostly prostitutes, whores, and those that suffered from nymphomania.

As the visit ended, he wished me well and flattered me by saying that I was a bright young man. To me, he wasn't crazy. It was ironic that he died of tuberculosis in this state facility. If he had been properly diagnosed, he could have been saved because there was another hospital about less than a mile as the crow flies to treat people with tuberculosis—The Uncas on the Thames.

To the reader, the hospital could and was probably used for medical experimentation on patients, and it is more than likely that some suffered cruel and unusual punishment. You be the judge, reader, of this very interesting institution and the reports.

The following document (author wishing to be unknown) has a lot of errors and is as I received it. I felt it was important to get another view on the issue in his own words.

The 60s

I was bom in 1956, a time when life was different. We always played outside and had few worries. I went to Saint Patrick's Catholic School in Norwich, Connecticut. I discovered early on that there was a separation of culture. I was Italian, so while I was in the 4th grade I was able to go to Delia's and eat a grinder for lunch. There was an Italian fest across Delia's neighborhood. Although my neighborhood was mostly Italian there was a mixed bag of all denominations. The downtown was still exciting. There were clothes shops and restaurants there. The Norwich Town Mall killed downtown. Women that drove could easily pull in and park and didn't have to worry about parallel parking. This was about the time when downtown became a dumping ground for Norwich State Hospital patients. There was an influx of patients who ended up there. The Waregan Hotel was their home. There they found their friends, package stores, and social services or welfare. The center of the city provided all the necessities. Metro area for people who needed assistance people could go to the mall instead. The Town let it turn out that way a place where a patient from Hartford, Vernon, wherever had it all.

The 70s

The 70s was still a downfall patient walking around scared people (women) from town. Many places were still there, cloth, food, restaurants, but decline continued caused by influx of patients parallel parking does not work for women. No insight to make it a destination the thought of college there did not happen, same with museum. The thought of removing a building does not work. It like having a missing front tooth. A parking lot needs a destination. Removal of the waterfront a big mistake (1950s). This was when the downtown was abandoned. Downtown needs an attraction. The scrap yard and police station is where it should come from. The thought of a college was also missed. The 70s had no one wanting to be there. Social service ended there and the town paid a price for it. The cost of the ccd is crazy. Should be one tax town. People find it hard to just pay the tax.

The 80s

Evacuation of downtown. Not much interesting except parking areas and parking lots. Buildings taken down. Lots put up with business moving out. Slum lords profit from patients. Downtown was taken advantage of.

Same in the 90s and the 20s

Downtown needs to be reinvented. Waterfront okay as long as odor from the sewer plant is controlled. The police department should go to Chestnut and North Franklin Street not Buckingham. Tax all the same. No ccd tax. Ethnic diversity accepted and it is what the town was built on. Incentives to move to downtown welcomed. Not to scare people off. The casino is at the doorstep. Time to work off their influx.

Authors notes: he meant the Wauregan Hotel; the CCD was the term given to the city consolidated city district, where if you lived within, your taxes would be higher as well as the "influx," which I believe he meant influence. Again, I left it the way he wrote it by his hand.

In the opinion column of The Bulletin on Sunday, April 26, 2019, was an article entitled <u>How Can Tolls and Taxes Reverse State's Decline?</u> by a writer named Chris Powell. Mr. Powell is a columnist for the Journal

Inquirer in Manchester. He ended his article by stating the following: "Showing Connecticut's decline, the state's economic and demographic data practically screams for challenging these policy premises, but there's too much profit for tod many people in continuing to do what drives the state down."

Again, the author's challenge is for future visitors and for the local residents to understand that we should feel welcomed when we travel to places (i.e., that mass transit should be inexpensive and efficient) and that decay and decline due to greed and stupidity should really cease to exist. But, reality, in the form of the decline of Norwich, shows just what Mr. Powell stated.

So, the challenge to you the reader is simple. See what remains of the Norwich State Hospital and the building of a theme park. Go to Norwich and note the decay. See the birth of people attempting to put the glow back into what was once called "The Rose of New England" with new businesses.

I have written this book to expose was actually happening at the hospital and the resultant effects on the city of Norwich it had when it closed down.

On 18 August 2019, at a press conference after two mass shootings, (one in Texas and the other in Ohio), President Donald Trump was asked what he intended to do about them. He basically put this whole issue of mental health out for the public by stating that. "It isn't the gun that pulls the trigger". He then mentioned seeing the effect of a mental institution closure when he lived in New York city and" We need to look at the issue of mental health" and mentioned that 92% of our institutions were shutdown to save the government money.

In summary best expressed by the Tea Party "83% of Americans blame mental health as a major issue. ((9/15/19) on a survey they took

Finally, for tourists I suggest looking at the Indian burial ground where the Masonic temple once stood, look at the Norwich city hall and its outside beauty of it all that and know that inside in a certain meeting room the city council members chairs are much higher than the public ones. Arrogance?? Explore, Ask residents, See the beautiful Uncas Leap Falls (when the river is high). Finally, explore the amazing contrast of a city trying to recover.

The following are more comments that I have added to entice you, the reader, to explore and to ponder.

16 November 1991
Dear Editor of the Bulletin,
Profit… A valuable gain.

Eminent Domain… The right of the Government to take private property for public use.

Citizens who oppose the Pequot expansion please understand what these words mean. I am sure that over ten million patrons and 10,000 employees have some say. Remember too that the tribe will have given the state over 200 million in taxes. They have already demonstrated the ability to "blend in" with their Foxwoods complex.

They need to expand and will do so despite your objections. Only the lawyers will profit from your good intentions.

Your blissful ignorance is not understanding profit is readily seen by the action of a certain town look in regards to a parking lot used by the employees. It now stands empty stark and ugly looking and is only giving those same townspeople minimum taxes in return. I say why not let the Pequots use the lot for a minimal fee until your illustrious leaders can get their act together and determine final use i.e., profit!

This sort of ignorance can readily be seen in downtown Norwich. Instead of providing for millions of tourists, traffic, and housing problems it instead has invested in grandiose schemes of a baseball stadium and now ice rink. All this while buildings stand empty and rot away!

Before you blame yourselves remember what happened to the great woolen industry thanks to both Federal and state government policies and interventions

Take charge of your destiny, people, and remember the words!

WILFRED ZINAVAGE
51 Hanover Versailles Road
Baltic, CT 06330
Phone: 860-822-1352 (after 5:00 p.m. please)

To: State of Connecticut, Environmental Committee
From: Linda Puetz, Sprague Board of Finance
Date: March 3, 1999

ACC SB 827
ACC HB 6006

Good morning my name is Linda Wilkinson Puetz. I reside in Hanover, a village in the Town of Sprague, Connecticut. I am here on behalf of ACC SB 827, ACC HB 6006, and any act concerning "Smart Growth" in Connecticut.

The headlines have become overwhelming… stadium to be built…stadium draws opposition… store owner fears closing business because Civic Center doesn't have enough foot traffic. The City of Norwich will exhaust you. The on again, off again Masonic Temple project, the on again, off again Wauregan Hotel, no hotel if the state doesn't fund a municipal parking lot… City Manager Talman needs more money from the state…the uptown, downtown of where the community college should be located…and the final straw the Mashantucket's pull out of the upscale, downscale, upscale of the Chelsea Exchange because it won't be a fiscal jackpot to them. You should see the hole they have left at the historic harbor.

All over the southeast the headlines continue in a similar fashion. Community Development president in dog fight with City manager… Fort Trumbull development plans displace residents… Griswold residents prefer renovation of historic town hall and vote for a park at the former Ashland Mill site… The Town of Sprague's historic center demise is kept a secret… Salem's historic corner store owner backs out after intervention by the Governor with DOT plans.

All these issues have a common thread, sprawl; a random scattering of development with no thought to what they mean for the environment or human community. This piecemeal planning has come from the top down. The community feels a sense of loss related to degradation of the environment and a sense of helplessness about various large scale urban problems.

To address these feelings the State of Connecticut must have a regional plan. A plan for people, a plan for neighborhood livability, a plan to support urban growth boundaries to prevent sprawl and most importantly a plan for its future. "Smart Growth' legislation can be the catalyst for this plan. A plan that will allow residents, neighborhoods, environmental groups, businesses, and local governments to be the author; to allow the community to keep intact the things it values the most and to shape infrastructure and other features offer opportunities to accommodate growth, with attention to compatibility with neighborhood character and values of those who live there.

"Smart Growth" will demand ingenious ways to revive troubled communities, reclaim Brownfields, remake cheap commercial strips, and forge regional alliances to help poorer communities. It will help design transportation that is transit oriented, redirect growth boundaries that protect greenspace and encourage Greenfield development. It will contain sprawl and revitalize our communities. It will put to rest the conflicts of the developers, the governments, the businesses and the communities.

"Smart Growth" is Connecticut's Field of Dreams. If enacted this legislation will make this administration's legacy not about a stadium, not about "Smart Growth", but about what counts most…the people of Connecticut. Thank you for your attention to this very important legislation.

The Norwich State Hospital Original Reports
June and July, 1953

SPECIAL THERAPEUTIC PROCEDURES
JUNE 1953

	Men	Women	Total
Shock Therapy:			
Electro-convulsive	55	66	121
Insulin Shock	26	34	60
Combined EST and Insulin	0	6	6
Antilustic Therapy:			
Penicillin	2	0	2
Endocrine Therapy:			
Regular Insulin	2	0	2
Protemine Zinc Insulin	5	18	23
H.P.H	0	1	1
Thyroid	0	1	1
Liver	0	1	1
Estrogenic	1	0	1
Parenteral Vitamins:			
Ferrocol	0	1	1
Unicaps	0	2	2
Ensolbec C	13	6	19
Vitamin B-12	0	1	1
Special Chemotherapy:			
Penicillin	47	47	94
Cortisone	1	0	1
Aureomycin	4	0	4
Streptomycin	3	3	6

	Men	Women	Total
Terramycin	4	4	8
Sulfa	0	1	1
Gantrisin	1	1	2
Streptomycin & PAS	33	12	45
INAH & PAS	1	5	6
Special Psychotheraphy:			
Group			
Number of Groups	1	0	1
Number of Patients	16	0	16
Number of Hours	7	0	7
Individual –			
Number of Patients	128	279	407
Number of Hours	615	475	1090
Narcotherapy:			
Sodium Amytal Interviews	1	2	3
Physiotherapy:			
Applications of Heat	15	1	16
Passive and Corrective Excercises	42	8	50
Total Number of EMPLOYEES treated in Physiotherapy	16	10	26
Whirlpool (hydro)	68	0	68
Vaccinations and Inoculations:			
Typhoid	39	0	39
Small Pox	24	0	24
__drotherapy:			
__ontinuous Tub:			
Number of Patients	15	20	35
Number of Hours	741 1/2	555-3/4	1,297
______ Sheet Packs:			
Number of Patients	14	148	162
Number of Packs	114	663	777
Number of Hours	342	1921	2,263
Special Protective and Supportive Procedures:			
Blood Transfusion	1	1	2
Clyses	15	6	21

	Men	Women	Total
Intravenous Feedings	1	5	6
__estraints:			
Sheets	1	47	48
Waist	2	0	2
Mittens	0	10	10
Wrist and Ankle	4	0	4
Wrist	4	4	8
Total Number of Hours	275 1/2	13,264	13539 1/2
__eclusion:			
Total Number of Patients	24	105	129
Total Number of Hours	1,705	11,618-3/4	13,323-3/4
TOTAL NUMBER OF PATIENTS RECEIVING TREATMENTS:	628	856	1,484

SPECIAL DIAGNOSTIC PROCEDURES		
JUNE 1953		
	Men	Women	Total
Electrocardiograph	13	35	48
Electro-encephalogram	20	15	35
Lumber Puncture	9	3	12

HYDROTHERAPHY
JUNE 1953

	Men	Women	Total
WET SHEET PACKS:			
Number of Packs	114	663	777
Number of Hours	342	1,921	2,263
Number of Patients	14	148	162
RESTRAINT:			
Number of Patients	11	61	72
Number of Hours	275 1/2	13,264	13539 1/2
Sheets	1	47	48
Waist	2	0	2
Mittens	0	10	10
Wrist and Ankle	4	0	4
Wrist	4	4	8
SECLUSION:			
Number of Patients	24	105	129
Number of Hours	1,705	11,618-3/4	13,323-3/4
HYDROTHERAPY:			
Number of Patients	15	20	35
Number of Hours	741 1/2	555-3/4	1,297

PHYSICIANS MONTHLY REPORT
JUNE 1953

A. Medical-Surgical (Employees)	Men	Women	Total
Number of Employees Treated	81	153	234
Number of Employees Treated	5	8	13
Number Hospital Days	19	27	46
Physical Examination of New Employees	11	11	22
Physical Re-examinations (food and milk handlers)	10	8	18
Compensation Forms	15	27	42
Typhoid Immunization	13	11	24
Total:	135	218	353

B. Medical—Surgical Outpatient Clinic (Patients)	Men	Women	Total
Number of Patients—Surgical	32	11	43
Number of Patients—Medical	13	22	35
Eye, Ear, Nose and Throat	8	12	20
Tumor Clinic	7	10	17
Gyn. Examinations	-	7	7
Total:	60	62	122

C. Consultation—Visiting Staff	Men	Women	Total
Ear, Nose and Throat (non-clinic cases)	3	-	3
Surgery	7	1	8
Orthopedics	1	1	2
Urology	1	-	1
Chiropody	36	72	108
Total:	48	74	122

SPECIAL SUMMARY ENTERIC SERVICE
JUNE 1953

Number of Typhoid Carriers6 (women)

SPECIAL PSYCHIATRIC EXAMINATION AND DIAGNOSTIC PROCEDURES
JUNE 1953

	Men	Women	Total
Routine Weekly Psychiatric Review Notes	146	106	252
Routine Monthly Psychiatric Review Notes	131	146	277
Routine Semi-Annual Psychiatric Review Notes	9	13	22
Routine Annual Psychiatric Review Notes	107	132	240
Number Cases Presented to General Staff Conference	1	3	4
Number Cases Presented for Consideration of Release	36	28	64
Letters Answered Reviewing Psychiatric Condition	78	43	121
Admission Mental Status Examinations	43	33	76

SPECIAL REPORT
JUNE 1953

	Number of Operations		
	Men	Women	Total
Major Surgical Procedures:			
Cholecysteotomy	1	-	1
Lobectomy, right lower lobe	1	-	1
Herniorrhaphy, right inguinal	3	-	3
Hemorrhoideotomy	1	-	1
Hysterectomy and Bilateral Salpino Oophorectomy	-	1	1
Total:	6	1	7
Minor Surgical Procedures:			
	Men	Women	Total
Bronchoscopy.	2	-	2
Cystoscopy	1	-	1
Incision and Drainage of Infection	7	4	11
Luetic Spinal Puncture	9	4	13
Removal of Callous	1	1	2
Removal of Foreign Bodies	1	1	2
Removal of Papilloma	1	-	1
Removal of Sebaceous Cyst	1	-	1
Removal of Splinter	-	2	2
Repair of Lacerations	5	3	8
Starnal Puncture	1	-	1
Thoracentesis	3	-	3
Total:	32	17	49
Fracture Treatment:			

	Men	Women	Total
Metatarsal, right. Cast Applied	1	-	1
Tibia, left. Cast Applied	1	-	1
Humerus, right. Cast Applied	1	-	1
Thumb, left. Plaster Splint	-	1	1
Total:	3	1	4

LABORATORY REPORT

JUNE 1953

Name of Test	Number of Tests
Urinalysis:	
Sugar	309
Routine	492
Acetone	22
Culture	1
Barbiturate	1
Hematology:	
Hemoglobin	232
R.B.C.	232
W.B.C.	234
Differential	234
Sedimentation Rate	17
Bleeding Time	2
Clotting Time	2
Cross Matching	17
Blood Typing	7
R.H. Factor	5
Culture—Blood	3
Blood Chemistry:	
Sugar	248
Urea Nitrogen	190
N.P.N	11
Creatinine	42
Total Protein	4
Albumin	4
Globulin	4
Cephalin Flocculation	3
Cholesterol	1
Van den Bergh	1

Name of Test	Number of Tests
Serology:	
Kolmer	6
V.D.R.L.	111
Spinal Fluids:	
Kolmer	11
Pandy	9
Cell Count	11
Colloidal Gold Curve	11
Chloride	3
Sugar	4
Total Protein	11
Stools:	
Culture	198
Occult Blood	2
Ova	3
Sputum:	
Culture	39
Smears	112
Sputum—contimed:	
Gastric Cultures	38
Total Number of Tests	2887
Total Number of Histology Slides	146

REPORT OF AUTOPSIES AND DEATHS
JUNE 1953

	Men	Women	Total	%
Number of Deaths	10	12	22	
Number of Autopsies	3	1	4	18%
Number of Medico-Legal Cases	3	3	6	

CAUSES OF DEATH AS SHOWN ON AUTOPSY REPORTS

Rocco George A-53-36 male.

Anatomical Diagnosis: Generalized Arteriosclerosis; Dilatation of the Ventricles of the Heart; endocarditis with Formation of Cardiac Mural. Thrombi; Old Healed Pleurisy; Old Infarcts of the Kidney; Moderate Hypertrophy of the Prostate; Chronic Passive Congestion of the Viscera.

Clinical Diagnosis: Acute Cardiac Dilatation; Chronic Endocarditis; Arteriosclerosis.

Mary Martinean A-53-37 female.

Anatomical Diagnosis: Generalized Arteriosclerosis; Hypertrophy and Dilatation of the Ventricles of the Heart; Chronic Pericarditia Senile Arteriosclerosis Kidnet; Hyphosis; Ascites; Chronic Passive Congestion of the Viscera.

Clinical Diagnosis: Acute Cardiac Dilatation; Arteriosclerotic Heart Disease.

George Getchill A-53-38 male.

Anatomical Diagnosis: Generalized Arteriosclerosis (aorta, coronary and cerebral arteries); Hypertrophy of the Ventricles of the Heart; Congestion and Emphysema of the Lungs; Senile Arteriosclerotic Kidneys; chronic Passive Congestion of the Viscara.

Clinical Diagnosis: Arteriosclerotic Heart Disease; Generalized Arteriosclerosis.

Edmond Deschamps A-53-39 male.

Anatomical Diagnosis: Bilateral Lober Pneumonia (left lung, both lobes, right lung, lower lobe); Obliterating Pericarditis; Moderate Arteriosclerosis (aorta, coronary arteries); Hypertrophy and Dilatation of the Ventricles of the Heart; Fatty Degeneration of the Liver; Hypoplasia of the Abdominal Aorta; Chronic Passive Congestion of the Viscera.

Clinical Diagnosis: Posterior Infarot of Myocarditis; Bronchopneumonia; Myocardial Insufficiency.

CAUSES OF DEATH AS SHOWN ON DEATH CERTIFICATES

		Age at Death
1.	Bronchopneumonia; Arteriosclerosis; Amputation, left midthigh	76
1.	Acute Cardiac Dilatation; Arteriosclerotic Heart Disease	72
1.	Recurrent Pneumonia; Arteriosclerotic Heart Disease; Gen. Arteriosclerosis	70
1.	Carebrovascular Accidents; Cerebral Arteriosclerosis; Gen. Arteriosclerosis	66
1.	Arteriosclerotic Cardiovascular Disease; Diabetes Mellitus	68
1.	Acute Cardiac Dilatation; Chronic Endocarditis; Arteriosclerosis	55
1.	Coronary Thrombosis; Arteriosclerotic Heart Disease	58
1.	Acute Cardiac Dilatation; Arteriosclerotic Heart Disease	65
1.	Pulmonary Embolus; Fracture, right femir; Generalized Arteriosclerosis	75
1.	Terminal Bronchopneumonia; Arteriosclerosis, generalized and advanced	66
1.	Pulmonary Tuberculosis; Chronic Myocarditis and Endocarditis	79
1.	Bronchopneumonia; Carcicoma of Extrinsic Larynx	59
1.	Acute Cardiac Dilatation; Art. Heart Disease	68
1.	Gangrene of left foot; Art. Heart Disease; Cerebral Arteriosclerosis	53
1.	Arteriosclerotic Heart Disease; Generalized Arteriosclerosis	78

1.	Posterior Infract of Nyocarditis; Bronchopneumonia; Myocarlial Insufficiency	41
1.	Hypostatic Pneumonia; Bronchial Asthma	48
1.	Bronchopneumonia; Metustatic Carcinoma of Lungs; Carcinoma of Rectum	50
1.	Myocardial Insufficiency; Arteriosclerotic Ht. Disease; Cerebral Art	85
1.	Myocardial Insufficiency, Generalized Arteriosclerosis; Art. Ht. Disease	89
1.	Cerebrovascular _______; generalized Arteriosclerosis	91
1.	One patient expired on placement at Convalescent Hospital	
Average Age at Death		671

REPORT OF
X-RAY DEPARTMENT

Part Examined	Examinations		Films
Abdomen	4		5
Ankle	8		12
Arm	7		11
Chest	313		318
Femur	1		1
Foot	5		6
G.I. Series, Stomach and Fluoroscopy	3		11
G.I. Series, Colon and Fluoroscopy	5		17
Hand	11		11
Hip, Routine	1		2
Jaw	1		2
Knee	7		11
Leg	4		5
Mastoids	1		8
Nose	2		4
Pelvis	9		11
Pyelogram, Intravenous	1		5
Ribs	2		3
Shoulder	8		19
Skull, routine	18		83
Spine, dorsal	36		36
Spine, lumber	8		19
Spine, Sacrum and Coccyx	4		8
Wrist	6		6
Total Patients Examined	394		
Total Number of Examinations		465	
Total Number of Film			614

SOCIAL SERVICE REPORT
JUNE 30, 1953

Case Count

Extended Visit	Male	Female	Total			
Carried Over	176	195	371			
Added During Month	19	25	44			
Total	195	220	415			
Closed						
Discharge of Patient	22	12	34			
Return of Patient	6	5	11			
Closed during month	28	17	45			
Total	167	203	370			
Family Care (Regular)						
Carried Over	8	10	18			
Added During Month	1	1	2			
Total	9	11	20			
Closed						
Extended Visit Granted	0	1	1			
Return of Patient	0	1	1			
Total	0	2	2			
CARRIED FORWARD				9	9	18
Family Care (Dr. Friedman's Convalescent Home)						
Carried Over				21	15	36
Added During Month				1	0	1

Total	22	15	37
Closed			
Extended Visit Granted	0	0	0
Return of Patient	2	0	0
Total	2	0	2
CARRIED FORWARD	20	15	35
Family Care (Golden Heights Chronic and Convalescent Hospital)			
Carried Over	6	19	25
Added During Month	0	1	1
Total	6	20	26
Closed			
Extended Visit Granted			0
Expired	0	1	1
Total	0	1	1
CARRIED FORWARD	6	19	25
Family Care ______ Chronic and ______ Hospital			
Carried Over	25	24	39
Added During Month	0	0	0
Total	25	24	39
Closed			
Extended Visit Granted	0	0	0
Return of Patient	0	0	0
Total	0	0	0
CARRIED FORWARD	25	14	39
GRAND TOTAL IN FAMILY CARE CONVAL. HOMES	51	48	99

Pre-Visit Studies						
Carried Over				6	3	9
Added During Month				1	6	7
Total				7	9	16
Closed						
Visit Granted				2	1	3
Visit Refused				2	0	2
Total				4	1	5
CARRIED FORWARD				3	8	11
2. Number of Interviews for						
Supervision of Patient on visit					10	
Supervision of patient in Family Care					39	
Pending Placement of Patient in Family Care					1	
Family Care Home Finding					0	
Psychiatric Social Histories					37	
Pre-Visit Studies					8	
Personal Services					30	
Total					125	
			Total	Grand Total		
3. Person Interviewed						
Patient			67			
Relative			51			
Collateral			7			
Total				125		
4. Place of Interview						
Hospital			80			
Field			45			
Total				125		

HARTFORD CLINIC		OUT PATIENT SERVICE			MONTH ENDING	
					30-Jun-53	
Caseload—Follow-up		New	Reopened		Total	
Cases carried over		132			132	
Added during month		12			12	
Total		144			144	
Closed during month		9			9	
Carried end of month		135			135	
Caseload—Treatment		New	Reopened		Total	
Cases carried over		15			15	
Added during month		3			3	
Total		18			18	
Closed during month		1			1	
Carried end of month		17			17	
Reason for Closure			Condition			
		Unimp	Imp	Much Imp	Rec'd	Total
No further treatment indicated						
Not amenable to treatment						
Referred to other agencies						
Hospitalized		2				2

HARTFORD CLINIC		OUT PATIENT SERVICE			MONTH ENDING	
Discharged from Visit			1	5		6
Follow-up to Treatment		2				2
						10
Source of Referral						
Patient						
Relative						
Hospital						
Doctor						
Social Agency						
Other	2					
Routine Follow-up	13					
Total	15					
Purpose of Interview			Person Seen			
		Pt.	Rel.		Total	
Follow-up						
Check-up		37	23		60	
Consultation		6	4		10	
Total		43	27		70	
Treatment		20	6		26	
Total Interviews		63	33		96	
Conferences with Other Agencies		2				
Psychological Test						
Telephone Calls		7				

HARTFORD CLINIC		OUT PATIENT SERVICE			MONTH ENDING	
Follow-up Appointments Made	69					
Kept	9					
Not kept but responded	21					
Not kept-no response	99					

OUT PATIENT SERVICE
BACKUS HOSPITAL CLINIC

Month Ending June 30, 1953
OCCUPATIONAL THERAPY REPORT
JUNE 1953

Caseload					
Cases Carried Over	42				
New Referrals	18				
Cases Re-opened	3				
Closed During Month	38				
Carried at End of Month	25				
Reasons for Closure		Condition			
		Unim proved	Im proved	Much Imp.	Reco vered
No further treatment indicated		-	4	6	1
Not emenable to specialized trtmnt		21	5	-	-
Referred to Other Agencies		-	-	-	-
Hospitalized		1	-	-	-

	Total: (38)	22	9	6	1
Sources of Referral		New		Re-opened	
Patient		2		3	
Relative		1		-	
Hospital		1		-	
Doctor		2		-	
Social Agency		12		-	
	Total	18		3	
Purpose of Interview					
Diagnostic Evaluation		31			
Treatment		84			
Relatives		9			
Total Number of Interviews		124			
Psychological Test				8	
Conference with Other Agencies				1	
Appointments:	Not kept but responded			2	
	Not kept, no response			5	
Psychiatric Reports				9	

REPORT OF THE HOSPITAL DENTIST
JUNE 1953

	TREATMENTS	PATIENTS
Dentures Repaired	7	7
Dentures Marked and Cleaned	36	22
Impressions for Dentures	2	1
Artificial Dentures	3	2
Examinations	70	70
Extractions:		
Novocaine	64	35
N-20	3	1
Root Canal Therapy	7	4
X-Rays:		
Intra-oral	25	12
Fillings	49	24
Prophylaxis	6	6
Treatments	24	19
Surgical Extractions	1	1
Total Number of Treatments	297	
Total Number of Patients		204

OCCUPATIONAL THERAPY REPORT
JUNE 1953

MEN'S ADMISSION SERVICE	
OCCUPATIONAL THERAPY SHOP	Average Daily Attendance 24
Chairs, refinished	12
Bookends, constructed, pairs	5
Ashtrays	2
Hardware cabinet, constructed	1
Bread cans, painted	2

OCCUPATIONAL THERAPY REPORT
JUNE 1953

WOMEN'S ADMISSION SERVICE	
OCCUPATIONAL THERAPY SHOP	Average Daily Attendance 32
Dresser Scarves	4
Table Mats	9
Colonial Mat	1
Chair Seat	1
Rugs	2
Potholders	9
Scarves	2

OCCUPATIONAL THERAPY REPORT
JUNE 1953

MEN'S OCCUPATIONAL THERAPY SHOP

	Average Daily Attendance	32
Ball; croquet striped, varnished		1
Basket; pharmacy type, constructed, varnished, lettered		1
Bed guard rails, repainted		9
Benches; small lawn, repaired, repainted		8
Benches, wood, repainted		2
Bird house repaired, stained		1
Board for clay cutting, constructed		1
Boxes; egg, constructed, painted, lettered		16
Box; file covered, constructed, varnished		2
Box; open file, constructed, varnished		2
Boxes; partitioned, constructed, varnished		2
Box; tool, constructed, varnished		1
Bulletin boards; constructed, painted, varnished		1
Cabinet; open file, constructed, varnished		1
Cabinet; record, constructed, varnished		1
Cans, low, painted		8
Cans; treated and painted		2
Cans; step-on, repainted		1
Chair; dining room, seat caned all refinished		1

Chair; lawn repaired, repainted		5
Chairs; metal, repainted		17
Chairs; metal and wood repainted		1
Chairs; plain ward, refinished		12
Chairs; plain ward, repainted		9
Compartment tray for desk drawer, constructed, varnished		1
Containers, flower, painted		3
Covers, rubber, lettered		2
Desk; constructed, shellacked, varnished		1
Frames; pictures, constructed, hellacked, varnished		24
Malletts, croquet, repaired, varnished		3
Mats; chair, hooked		7
Mats; table, hooked		2
Plates; tin, painted		4
Racks; book, constructed, varnished		2
Rack, large, constructed, painted		1
Rack; mop, constructed, painted		1
Rocker; metal, painted		1
Rocker; porch, back and seat caned, varnished		2
Rocker; porch, seat caned, varnished		2
Rug, knotted		1
Rugs, woven		8
Runner, woven		4
Signs, lettered, painted or varnished		4
Signs; with standard, constructed, lattered, varnished		2
Stepladders; constructed, painted		3
Stools; constructed, varnished, lettered		12
Table; bridge, constructed, painted		1
Tables; small, painted		2
Tables; small, constructed, paint		2

Tables; small with shelf, constructed, varnished		2
Trays; folding, constructed, painted		6
Tray; medication, constructed, varnished		1
Wastebaskets; painted, decorated		23
Wickets; croquet, painted, sets		

OCCUPATIONAL THERAPY REPORT
JUNE 1953

SEWING ROOM		Average Daily Attendance 74
NEW ARTICLES		
Aprons, cafeteria, men's 15"		68
Aprons, cafeteria, men's 30"		42
Aprons, kitchen, bib		38
Aprons, rubber		54
Covers, bed pan		83
Covers, mattress 30"		29
Covers, mattress 36"		34
Covers, wrapper		18
Curtains, shower		2
Dresses, print		170
Dresses, hercutex swirl		43
Draperies, pairs		6
Gowns, night		122
Gowns, nurses		21
Pajamas, women's pairs		41
Pajamas, men's pairs		36
Pants, altered		25
Pillow cases, rubber		100
Sheets, pack		6
Sheets, safty, hydrotherapy		5
Hammocks, hydrotherapy		5
Slips		342
Uniforms, _____tered		10
	TOTAL	1300

MENDED ARTICLES			
Aprons	6	Goens, night	1
Awnings	5	Hammocks, hydro	1
Bags, Laundry	19	Harnesses	101
Bathrobes	177	Overalls	996
Bedjackets	30	Pajama coats	2
Bedspreads	166	Pants	333
Blankets	63	Pants, cafeteria	20
Blouses, strong	53	Pillow cases	18
Camisole	1	Scarf, bureau	1
Coats, suit	12	Sheets	762
Coveralls	9	Sheets, Hydro	8
Dresses, hercutex, regular	2	Shirts, top	20
Dresses, print	17	Slacks	36
Dresses, swirl	89	Slips	8
Dropcloth, painters	35	Suit, baseball	1
Flags	6	Sweaters	36
Floorpads	3	Underwear	44
Gowns, johnnie coats	628		
		TOTAL	3709

OCCUPATIONAL THERAPY REPORT
JUNE 1953

WOMEN'S OCCUPATIONAL THERAPY SHOP	Average Daily Attendance 29
Altar Cloths with wide crocheted edgings	3
Bedside Screen Curtains	18
Curtains, made, pairs	122
Curtains tiebacks, sewn, pairs	120
Curtain tiebacks, crocheted, pairs	36
Dish towels, hemmed	550
Hand towels, hemmed	472
Hooked seat covers, lined	9
Mouth gags	1360
Stockings, mended, pairs	413
Table Runners, embroidered, edges crocheted	12
Tapes sewn on syringe covers	96
Wash Cloths, hemmed	220
BRYAN OCCUPATIONAL THERAPY SHOP	Average Daily Attendance 46
Socks Mended, pairs	610
Ear Tabs	1200
Dresses Mended	102
Towels, dish	100
Doilies, crocheted	9
Strips cut	
Strips sewn	

BELL OCCUPATIONAL THERAPY SHOP	Average Daily Attendance 18
Crocheted piece	1
Rug, rag	1
Rug, crocheted, roving	1
Rug, hooked	1
Scarves, bedside table	4
Scarves, dresser	3
Vanity set (3 pc.)	1
Newspaper covers colored	
Decorations for clubhouse party	

OCCUPATIONAL THERAPY REPORT
JUNE 1953

SHOE SHOP	Average Daily Attendance 7
Belts repaired	2
Clocks repaired	2
Shoes Exchanged, pairs	15
Repaired, Half Soles, pairs	20
Heeled, Composition, pairs	24
Rubber, pairs	37
Heel Linings, pairs	11
Pads, pairs	25
Insoles, pairs	2
Plates, pairs	3
Paten and sewn, pairs	41
Restitch Soles, pairs	1
Basketball sewn	1
Repair skate straps	5
Repair baseball bases	3
UPHOLSTERY SHOP	Average Daily Attendance 8
Chairs, refinished	2
Chairs, repaired bottom	1
Mattresses, constructed	69
Shades, window, repaired	21
Table, refinished	1
Venetian Blinds, repaired	10

MEN'S OCCUPATIONAL THERAPY PRINT SHOP	
Cards our only	108
Pads Stapled	246
Pads Glued	596
Pads Glued (Used paper)	270
Manifold	532
Assembled (Multigraph Impressions)	459
(Duplicating Impressions)	2020
Triple Holes Punched (Multigraph Impressions)	6200
Double Holes Punched (Multigraph Impressions)	15400
Assembled & Stapled (Multigraph Impressions)	10000
(Duplicating Impressions)	1200
Duplicating Impressions	16525
Printing Impressions	37368
Multigraph Impressions	72645

OCCUPATIONAL THERAPY REPORT
JUNE 1953

OCCUPATIONAL THERAPY MENDING ROOM	
BELL BUILDING	Average Daily Attendance 29
Aprons	1
Bathrobes	25
Blouses	39
Blouses, strong	2
Dresses	3677
Gowns, doctors	292
Gowns, nurses	60
Pajama coats	72
Pajama pants	121
Pants	17
Shirts, top	1060
Shorts	330
Skirts	21
Slacks, farmerette	3
Slips	1195
Sweaters	8
Underwear, female	693
Union suits	159
Underdrawers	1
Undershirts	147
OCCUPATIONAL THERAPY	
WARD PROJECTS	

LIPPITT 3:	
4"x4" Gauze Compresses	958 dz.
ABD. Pads	498 dz.
LIPPITT 4:	
2"x2" Gauze Compresses	732 dz.
4"x4" Gauze Compresses	166 dz.
STRIBLING:	
Chairs sanded	6
Beds sanded	4

OCCUPATIONAL THERAPY REPORT
JUNE 1953

RECREATIONAL THERAPY REPORT		
	No.	Average
	Times	Attendance
Classes in roller skating	70	41
Moving Pictures (Theatre)	8	421
Lawn Games	12	21

June 5, 1953. The Cootiettes, Veterans of Foreign Wars Auxiliary, gave a party for 67 veterans at the clubhouse this afternoon. The patients participated in word games. Refreshments and cigarettes were served by the auxiliary members, after which all participated in group singing.

June 9, 1953. There were 80 veterans in attendance at a party this afternoon at the clubhouse, sponsored by the American Legion Auxiliary of Baltic. Games were enjoyed, and following entertainment, refreshments of sandwiches, cookies, ice cream, coffee, and cigarettes were served by the ladies of the auxiliary.

June 16, 1953. The Veterans of Foreign Wars Auxiliary of New London gave a party for 87 veteran at the clubhouse. Entertainment consisted of an observation quiz, a true and false contest, and a musical quiz. Refreshments and cigarettes were served by Mrs.

Mary Murphy and her committee, after which dancing was enjoyed.

	No.	Average
Clubhouse Activities:	Times	Attendance
Bell	5	40
Butler	1	8
Mitchell	4	29
Woodward	1	14
Brigham	5	25
Stribling	2	16
Gallup	4	31
Earle	1	12
Bingo Parties:		
Salmon 1	5	
Salmon 11	5	
Gallup	3	
Stribling 1	4	
Stribling 11	4	
White	4	
Earle	4	

OCCUPATIONAL THERAPY REPORT
JUNE 1953

RECREATIONAL THERAPY REPORT (CONTINUED)

		No. Times	Average Attendance
Moving Pictures shown on wards:			
Seymour 1		4	34
Seymour 3		4	38
White		5	100
Galt		5	54
Kirkbride 3		5	112
Kirkbride 1		5	90
Lippitt 4		5	10
Gallup 2		4	51
Salmon 2		4	32
Salmon 1		4	42
Seymour 2		4	42
Seymour 4		4	30
Lippitt 4		5	20
Ray		5	90
Dix		5	44
Bell		4	51
Mitchell		4	20
Cutter		4	120
Bryan		4	125
CHOIR REHEARSALS:		5	20
Choir (Sundays)		3	20
Group singing (Woodward, Stedman)		4	

RELIGIOUS SERVICES:			
Protestant Services June 7, 14, 21, 28			
Catholic Services June 7, 14, 21, 28			
Protestant Servies held on wards:			
Bryan	June 7		
Ray 2 & 3	14		
Seymour 2, 3 & 4	28		
KirkBride	21		
Salmon 1 & 2 Alternate	Sunday		

OCCUPATIONAL THERAPY REPORT
JUNE 1953

NORWICH STATE HOSPITAL
WOMEN'S AUXILIARY

On June 4, members of the Women's Auxiliary, Mrs. Tingley, Mrs. Brambilla, Mrs. Sandberg, Mrs. Lynch, and Mrs. Stoudt visited patients in the Seymour Building.

OCCUPATIONAL THERAPY REPORT
JUNE 1953

On June 24, four patients from the Women's Admission Service accompanied by an employee, attended the matinee performance of "Kiss and Tell", starring Margaret O'Brien, at the Norwich Summer Theatre. The tickets were made available to our patients through the courtesy of the Norwich College Club and Mr. Herbert Kneeter, manager of the Norwich Summer Theater.

OCCUPATIONAL THERAPY REPORT
JUNE 1953

On June 3, Occupational Therapy students from the Ohio State University, University of Illinois, Columbia University, and the Philadelphia School of Occupational Therapy visited the Mansfield state Training School and Hospital.

On June 24, Miss Patricia Susan Maguire, an English Exchange student from the Philadelphia School of Occupational Therapy completed her clinical affiliation at this hospital.

The following Occupational Therapy students began their clinical affiliation in psychiatry. June 1, Ohio State University students, the Misses Susan Lehman, Arden Pfouts; Columbia University, the Misses Audrey Smith, Elsie Doran; June 8, Mount Mary College, Miss Margaret M. Nilles June 15, University of Kansas, the Misses Barbara Elam, Mary Snead, Carolyn Blouch, Lyle Mesker, and Rose Marie Novotny; June 29, University of Illinois, the Misses Joy Anderson and Jean Prebis Ohio State University, the Misses Nona Toops and Lena Futhey; Philadelphia School of Occupational Therapy. Miss Naomi J. Young.

OCCUPATIONAL THERAPY REPORT
JUNE 1953

REPORT ON INDUSTRY

Main Kitchen	36
Dining Room, Congregate	37
Dining Room, Employees	6
Laundry	34
Engineering Department	13
Housekeeping	65
Store Room	5
Farm and Barns	64
Others	319
	579
Ward Work	322
Ward Classes	18

OCCUPATIONAL THERAPY REPORT
REPORT OF THE GENERAL LIBRARY
JUNE 1, 1953–JULY 1, 1953

TOTAL CIRCULATION 4313
TOTAL ATTENDANCE 1288

CIRCULATION IN THE LIBRARY:	
Books issued to patients	380
Books issued to employees	2
Magazines issued	840
Newspapers issued	319
Puzzles issued	96
CIRCULATION ON WARDS:	
Books issued	72
Magazines distributed	2539
Newspapers distributed	76
Puzzles distributed	96
READING ROOM ATTENDANCE	
Ward groups	123
General Attendance	1165
MAGAZINES RECEIVED:	
Subscriptions	20
No. received on subscription	35
No. gift magazines	807

BOOKS RECEIVED:	
Gifts	545
Purchased	none
ACCOUNTING REPORT:	
No. books catalogued	2452
No. new books added	50
No. books lost/destroyed	36
No. books in Patient's Library	4266
No. books in Seymour Library	487
No. books in Mitchell Library	79
No. books in Gallup Library	124
No. books in Bell Library	139
No. books in Bryan Library	44
TOTAL NUMBER OF BOOKS	5139

MEDICAL LIBRARY MONTHLY REPORT JUNE 1953

Number of books in library	4122
Number of books added	6
Total number of books in library	4128
Number of books circulated	317
Number of journals subscribed to	92
Number of journals received	101
Number of journals circulated	86
Interlibrary Loans	6
Material from MLA Exchange	2

Of the 6 books added to the Library in June, 1 was a replacement of a lost book, and the others were gifts.

	JUNE CIRCULATION
Year	Books and Journals
1951	308
1952	310 Increase 2
1953	403 Increase 93

ACCIDENT REPORT
JUNE, 1953

MEN	No.	WOMEN	No.
Lippitt	2	Lippit	2
Seymour	0	Seymour	2
Salmon	1	Awl	5
Brigham	5	Bell	23
White	18	Cutter	22
Stribling	4	Dix	8
Earle	4	Butler	10
Galt	6	Woodward	7
		Stedman	9
Gallup	28	Mitchelle	35
		Bryan	3
Kirkbride	12	Ray	29
		Sewing Room	2
Galt O.T. Shop	0	Beauty Salon	6
Total	80	Total	163

ANALYSIS OF ACCIDENTS

CAUSE OF ACCIDENTS	No Injury	Minor	Major
Cuts:			
Metal		5	
Falls:			
General	5	47	
Convulsive Seizures		8	
Quarrels Between Patients	3	47	
Unprovoked attacks	1	41	
Self-inflicted		15	
Collision	1	20	
Recreational Activity		4	
Industrial Activity		8	
Resistiveness to Routine Care		4	
Burns		11	
Combined Irritative Treatment		2	
Undetermined		20	
Pathological			1
Total	10	232	1

HOSPITAL CHAPLAIN'S REPORT
JUNE 1953
(PROTESTANT)

I. The Ministry of Worship:		
1. Total Number of Worship Services Conducted	17	
1. Average Attendance at these 17 Worship Services	1421	
1. Average Attendance per Sunday (Theatre)	178	
1. Number of Ward Services (Infirmaries and Prison Wards)	13	
1. Total Attendance at these 13 Ward Serices	707	
1. Total Number of Sermons Preached (Chaplain and Resident)	3	
II. The Sacramental Ministry:		
1. Number of Holy Communion Services Conducted	1	
1. Total Attendance at this Holy Communion Service	176	
1. Total Receiving Holy Communion	74	
III. The Pastoral Ministry—To Patients (Chaplain and Resident)		
1. Initial Religious Interviews with Newly Admitted Patients	8	

1.	Calls to Patients on the Danger List	18	
1.	All other Patients Visits	46	
1.	Interviews with Relatives of Patients	1	
1.	Total Hours (approximate) Patient Visits and Interviews	29	
IV. Hospital Teachings:			
1.	The Clinical Pastoral Training of Theological Students and Clergy:		
a.	Number of Students in Training	7	
a.	Chaplain's Conferences with Resident	13	(22 hours)
a.	Chaplain's Conferences with other Students	9	(11 hours)
a.	Resident's Conferences with students	7	(18 hours)
a.	Seminars led by Chaplain	8	(13 hours)
a.	Seminars led by Resident	5	(8 hours)

PUBLIC RELATIONS
JUNE 1953

MEETINGS ATTENDED:

June 2, 1953—Dr. Ronald h. Kettle attended a meeting of the Seminar Committee of Postgraduate Studies in Psychiatric and Neurology held in Middletown.

June 2, 1953—Mrs. Gusbee and Mrs. Wilson, Assistant Directors of Nursing, attended a meeting at the Grace-New Haven Community Hospital of the administrative section of the Connecticut State Nurses Association.

June 4, 1953—Drs. Steinecke and Doerr attended the neuropsychiatric section of the American Medical Association Meeting at the Hotel New Yorker in New York City on this date.

June 10 and 11, 1953—Miss. Shields, Nursing Education Director, met with the faculties of St. Joseph College and St. Frances Hospital in Hartford, and the New Britain General Hospital in New Britain.

June 11, 1953—Mr. Capon, Social Service Director, attended a meeting of the Norwich Health and Welfare council on this date.

June 18, 1953—Dr. Kettle attended the Monthly Meeting of the Personnel Advisory Committee at Hartford.

June 18, 1953—Mrs. Sauber of the Social Service Department attended the meeting of the United Workers held in Norwich on this date.

June 23, 1953—Mrs. Sauber and Mr. Melican (Social Service) attended the Annual Meeting of the Connecticut Association for Mental Hygiene. The meeting was held in New Britain.

LECTURE ATTENDED:

June 1, 1953—Doctors Doerr, Hennighan and Hooker attended a lecture at the Institute of Living in Hartford. Dr. Gabriel Langfeldt, Professor of Pschiatry and Superintendent of the Psychiatric Clinic at the University of Oslo, lectured on "Diagnosis and Prognosis in Schizophrenia."

INSTITUTE ATTENDED:

June 1, 1953—Mrs. Riden, Clinical Instructor, attended a one day institute on Nursing Care in Poliomyelitis in Hartford.

NATIONAL CONFERENCE:

May 31 to June 4, 1953, Mr. Capon attended the National Conference of Social Work in Clevaland, Ohio.

On June 26, 1953, Miss Eloise Shields sailed on the SS *Argentine* for Rio de Janeiro where she will attend the meetings of the International Council of Nurses. From Brazil, she will go to Lima, Peru where she will attend the meeting of the World Federation of Mental Health. She has been invited to serve as Psychiatric Nurse-Consultant for this Group.

TALK BY ASSISTANT SUPERINTENDENT:

On June 9, Dr. Conrad Ranger, assistant superintendent, gave a talk on the social aspects of the personality to a medical group at Manchester, New Hampshire.

BOOKS REVIEWED:

The following books were reviewed for the Boston Medical Library, the reviews to be published in *The New England Journal of Medicine*:

- The Superego (E. Bergler) Reviewed by Dr. J. Wright.
- Presciption for Rebellion (R. Lindner) Reviewed by. Dr. I. Brown.

COMMUNITY RELATIONSHIPS REPORTED BY HOSPITAL CHAPLAIN:

Address Related to Chaplain's Work

June 14. Men's Corporate Communion Breakfast, Christ Church, Norwich (Chaplain)

June 14. Baptist Youth Fellowship, Norwich. (Address by Chaplain Resident)

June 16. Lutheran Brotherhood, First Lutheran Church in Norwich (Resident)

Assistance in Community Churches

Mr. Zimmerman, hospital chaplain, assisted in four services at Christ's Church in Norwich on June 7, June 14, June 21 and June 28.

Professional Meetings Attended

June 19. Board of Governors, Council for Clinical Training, New York City

June 29. Social Service Agency Visits, Hartford (entire training group)

84 EMPLOYEES ENTERED THE SERVICE DURING JUNE 1953

NAME	POSITION	DATE
Richard Siragusa	Farmhand	6/1/1953
Susan Lehman	Student Nurse (O.T.)	6/1/1953
Elsie Doran	Student Nurse (O.T.)	6/1/1953
Audrey Smith	Student Nurse (O.T.)	6/1/1953
Arden Pfouts	Student Nurse (O.T.)	6/1/1953
Gordon Lunt	Psychiatric Aide	6/2/1953
Lillie Howard, Rein.*	Psychiatric Aide	6/2/1953
Emil Labant	Psychiatric Aide	6/2/1953
Joseph Kobelski	Institution Helper	6/3/1953
Edward Miller, M.D.	Resident (Psy.)	6/3/1953
Helen McMullan, Rein.*	Tel. Operator	6/3/1953
Anthony Angelo, Rein.*	Psychiatric Aide	6/8/1953
Walter C. Bruschi, M. D.	Resident (Psy.)	6/8/1953
Raymond A. Guertin	Psychiatric Aide	6/8/1953
Margaret M. Nilles	Student Nurse (O.T.)	6/8/1953
Flecher Parker	Student Nurse (Theology)	6/8/1953
Samuel Vanculin		6/8/1953
Claud W. Behn, Jr.		6/8/1953
Charles A Horn		6/8/1953
Robert W. Jahns		6/9/1953
Kenneth E. Spilman		6/9/1953
George H. Cochran, Rein.*	Psychiatric Aide	6/10/1953
Rose-Alice Lemieux	Psychiatric Aide	6/10/1953
Margaret Renshaw	Psychiatric Aide	6/11/1953
Robin Mitchell	Psychiatric Aide	6/15/1953
Barbara Elam	Student Nurse (O.T.)	6/15/1953
Carolyn Blouch		6/15/1953
Lyle Mesker		6/15/1953
Rose Novotny		6/15/1953

NAME	POSITION	DATE
Mary Snead		6/15/1953
Marjorie Storms	Student Nurse	6/15/1953
Barbara Thompson		6/15/1953
Faye Evans		6/15/1953
Carol Killeen		6/15/1953
Gloria Lutsky		6/15/1953
Dorothy Janaites		6/15/1953
Marjorie Kayeski		6/15/1953
Marion Keene		6/15/1953
Marion Nodwell		6/15/1953
Pauline Rosys		6/15/1953
Carol Bourgeois		6/15/1953
Eleanor Brendel		6/15/1953
Rose Collins		6/15/1953
Beverly Deshefy		6/15/1953
Marie Doran		6/15/1953
Frances Genovese		6/15/1953
Margaret Hurley		6/15/1953
Glenna M. Jacobs		6/15/1953
Sylvia Johnstone		6/15/1953
Theresa Lemieux		6/15/1953
Donna Lorusso		6/15/1953
Jocephine Notaro		6/15/1953
Ruth P. O'Neil	Student Nurse	6/15/1953
Florence Slovitski		6/15/1953
Marjorie Bliss		6/15/1953
Mary-Ellen Bruno		6/15/1953
Doris Byers		6/15/1953
Maureen Daley		6/15/1953
Laurel Christman		6/15/1953
LaVerne Fakkema		6/15/1953
Rhoda Kaplan		6/15/1953
Margaretta Madden		6/15/1953
Constane Sturim		6/15/1953
Marcy Spinnato	Guard Attendant	6/16/1953
Rudolph Graska	Psychiatric Aide	6/16/1953
Alfred Staebner	Psychiatric Aide	6/17/1953
Robert Deveau	Psychiatric Aide	6/17/1953

NAME	POSITION	DATE
Dorothy Hartson, Rein.*	Psychiatric Aide	6/17/1953
Anne Lyman, Rein.*	Psychiatric Aide	6/17/1953
Charles Allen	Psychiatric Aide	6/22/1953
Beatrice McLean	Psychiatric Aide	6/24/1953
Emma Kirkman	Institution Helper	6/25/1953
Nancy Dwinell	Psychiatric Aide	6/26/1953
Renold Boudreau	Institution Helper	6/29/1953
Charles Kostelos	Institution Helper	6/29/1953
Elizabeth Griswold	Psychiatric Aide	6/29/1953
Judith Colpek	Psychiatric Aide	6/29/1953
Jean McRee, M. D.	Asst. Physician	6/29/1953
Jay Anderson	Student Nurse (O.T.)	6/29/1953
Lena Futhey		6/29/1953
Jean Prebis		6/29/1953
Nona Toops		6/29/1953
J. Naomi Young		6/29/1953

*Former Employee—Reinstated

49 EMPLOYEES LEFT THE SERVICE DURING JUNE 1953

NAME	POSITION	ACTION	DATE
Ruth Gebbie	Psychiatric Aide	TRNS	6/5/1953
Angela L. Jorsz	Psychiatric Aide	RES	6/6/1953
Irwin Rothman	Psychiatric Aide	RES	6/7/53 Noon
Arthur Hinse	Psychiatric Aide	LWN	6/7/1953
Lucy White	Psychiatric Aide	RES	6/7/1953
Ida May Jones	Psychiatric Aide	RES	6/9/53 Noon
Theresa Buechse	Psychiatric Aide	RES	6/9/1953
Nancy Holmberg	Student Nurse	TIME EXPIRED	6/15/1953
Pauline Mitchell			6/15/1953
Diana Hodge			6/15/1953
Velma Travers			6/15/1953
Rosemarie Caetano			6/18/1953

2 EMPLOYEES REASSIGNED DURING DURING JUNE 1953

NAME	POSITION FROM	POSITION TO	DATE
Norman Sewart	Inst. Helper	Cook	6/1/53
Rene Gauvin	Inst. Helper	Cook	6/2/53

SICK TIME
JUNE 1953

DEPARTMENT	NAME	POSITION	NO. OF DAYS
Business Office	Dix, Pauline	Telephone Operator	22
	MoCrohan, Nora	Clerk, Grade II	1
Central Clo. Room	Burgess, Anna	Seamstress	2
	Conway, Anna	Clo. Caretaker	1
	Roy, Margaret	Clo. Caretaker	1
	Schrier, Helen	Stores Clerk	1
	Soboleski, Catherine	Clo. Caretaker	1
	Sposato, Frank	Clo. Caretaker	1
Clin. Rec. Off.	Brennan. Jeanette	Steno., Grade II	1
Cong. Din. Room	Riccio, Harry	Inst. Helper	1
Dental	McCormick, Thomas	Senior Inst. Dentist	7 ½
Dietary	Chabotte, Samuel	Inst. Helper	4
	Duquette, Jennie	Din. Room Supv.	6
	Gauthier, Theresa	Inst. Helper	1
	Hayes, Ruth	Din. Room Supv.	1
	Lenkiewics, Felix	Cook	1
	Moran, Grace	Din. Room Supv.	15
Farm	Kudlach, Gasper	Farmhand	4
Housekeeping	Campey, Dorothy	Inst. Helper	½

DEPARTMENT	NAME	POSITION	NO. OF DAYS
	McMullen, Helen	Inst. Helper	4
	Pierce, Marie	Inst. Helper (Comp.)	6
	Quinn, Kathryn	Housekeeper	2
	Thompson, Anna Mae	Inst. Helper	2
Laboratory	Horris, Ann	Lab. Helper (Comp.)	30
Laundry	Aldi, Arthur	Cleaner	1
	Aubin, Paul	Laundry Supr.	2
	Gauthier, Edith	Laundry Worker	2
	Gromko, Anthony	Laundry Worker	2
	Hoxsie, David	Laundry Worker	1
	Kasansky, Meriam	Laundry Worker (Comp.)	30
	Lane, Thomas	Laundry Worker	1
	Lukaszewicz, Jeanne	Laundry Worker	1
	Morey, Yvette	Laundry Worker	1
	Pineault, Aline	Laundry Worker	2
	Ponatisten, Margaret	Laundry Worker	1
	Rec, Thomas	Laundry Worker	½
	Robert, Elsie	Laundry Worker	2
	Scott, Ida	Laundry Worker	1
	Steinman, Aaron	Laundry Worker	1
	Tedesco, Raffaelo	Laundry Worker	1 ½
	Ruth DeForge	Laundry Worker	1
Main Kitchen	Fratoni, Paul	Cook	4
	Lapre, Francer	Inst. Helper	6
	Nowakowski, Charles	Cook	3
	Redding, James	Cook	6
	Torrance, Frederick	Head Cook	1
	Tusia, Frank	Inst. Helper	5

DEPARTMENT	NAME	POSITION	NO. OF DAYS
Maintenace	Huntington, Cha___ing	Stat. Engineer	1
	Korab, Albert	Stat. Engineer (Comp.)	24
	Lamon, Charles	Steam Fireman	½
	Nowakowskie, Vincent	Skld. Trdsm	1
	Urban, Walter	Skld. Trdsm	1
Medical	Boyle, Desmond, M.D.	Sr. Resident (Psy.)	2
	Doerr, William, M. D.	Asst. Physician	1
Nursing Office	McClafferty, Helen	Nurse Clin. Instr.	2
Occup. Therapy	Cloutier, Blanche	Therapy Aide	7 ½
	Elliot, Peggy	Storekeeper (Canteen)	1
	Evert, Peggy	Occup. Therap. (Comp.)	30
	Joss, Mark K.	Occup. Therapist	½
	Kosoinski, Joseph	Therapy Aide	3
	Linda, Olga	Psychiatric Aide	1
Prison Ward	Barton, James	Guard Attendant	1
	Leone, Umbert	Guard Attendant	1
	Looby, Maurice	Chg. Guard Att.	12
Psychology	Chornoby, Micalena	Clerk, Gr. II	1
	Scales, Margaret	Clin. Psychologist	1
Nursing Service	Adams, Robert	Psychiatric Aide	1
	Bence, Pauline	Grad. Nurse	1
	Biedera, Sophie	Psychiatric Aide	1
	Blanchard, Joseph	Psy. Aide (Comp.)	21
	Blanchard, Susane	Graduate Nurse	2
	Bohara, Nellie	Psychiatric Aide	1

DEPARTMENT	NAME	POSITION	NO. OF DAYS
	Bolton, Marion	Psychiatric Aide	1
	Boudreau, Robert	Psychiatric Aide	3
	Bouthillier, Helen	Psychiatric Aide	5
	Brouillard, Mary	Psychiatric Aide	1
	Brown, Carole	Psy. Aide (Comp.)	11
	Brown, Carole	Psychiatric Aide	½
	Brown, Margaret	Charge Aide (Psy.)	1
	Brown, Kartina	Psychiatric Aide	1
	Burke, Margaret	Psychiatric Aide	1
	Burke, Mary	ChargeAide(Psy.) (Comp.)	30
	Butler, Anna	Charge Nurse	1
	Cadey, Delia	Psychiatric Aide	8
	Callahan, Frederick	Psychiatric Aide	2
	Caplet, Lorraine	Psychiatric Aide (Comp.)	5
	Caplet, Lorraine	Psychiatric Aide	1
	Carter, Delphinoa	Psychiatric Aide	1
	Chabot, Lucy	Psychiatric Aide	2
	Charron, Anne	Psychiatric Aide	1
	Chester, Frank	Psychiatric Aide	3
	Cloud, Victoria	Psychiatric Aide	2
	Coman, Herbert	Psychiatric Aide	1
	Cook, Elizabeth	Psychiatric Aide	1
	Cooley, Estelle	Psychiatric Aide	1
	Cooney, John	Psychiatric Aide	1
	Cote, Helen	Psychiatric Aide	1
Nursing Service	Couto, Ralph	Psychiatric Aide	1
	Cross, Emily	Charge Aide (Psy.)	1
	Crumley, Lillian	Psychiatric Aide	1
	Dabrowski, Frances	Psychiatric Aide	1
	Davis, Doris	Psychiatric Aide	1
	Davis, Ermoline	Psychiatric Aide	1
	Dayon, Dora	Psychiatric Aide	9

DEPARTMENT	NAME	POSITION	NO. OF DAYS
	Delmonte, Katherine	Psychiatric Aide (Comp.)	30
	Dennis, Annie	Psychiatric Aide	1
	Dennis, Everett	Psychiatric Aide	1
	Discoe, Carmella	Charge Nurse	1
	Donvan, Mildred	Psychiatric Aide	1
	Dorsey, Barbara	Psychiatric Aide	1
	Downing, Ernest	Psychiatric Aide	1 1/2
	Durand, John	Psychiatric Aide	1
	Durfee, Douglas	Psychiatric Aide (Comp.)	30
	Duro, Elmer	Psychiatric Aide	2
	Elton, Bertram	Psychiatric Aide	1
	Ferriter, Mary	Charge Aide (Psy.)	3
	Fish, Marjorie	Psychiatric Aide	1
	Flynn, Rose	Charge Aide (Psy.)	1
	Gagliardo, Frank	Psychiatric Aide	1
	Gagnon, Loretta	Psychiatric Aide	1
	Garey, Jeanne	Psychiatric Aide	1
	Garrow, Marjorie	Psychiatric Aide	1
	Gionet, Agnes	Psychiatric Aide	1
	Gionet, Annobert	Psychiatric Aide	2
	Gionet, Norman	Psychiatric Aide	2
	Gonzales, Angelo	Psychiatric Aide	4
	Green, Claree	Psychiatric Aide	2
	Greenwood, Beverly	Psychiatric Aide	1
	Greenwood, Phyllis	Psychiatric Aide	½
	Grenier, William	Psychiatric Aide (Comp.)	9
	Guyot, Louis	Psychiatric Aide	1
	Hayes, Margaret	Psychiatric Aide	2
	Hebert, Laurell	Graduate Nurse	2
	Hildebrand, Augusta	Charge Aide (Psy.)	2
	Inch, Adele	Charge Nurse	3

DEPARTMENT	NAME	POSITION	NO. OF DAYS
	Jaroch, Jean	Charge Nurse	1
	Jeanotte, Ernest	Psychiatric Aide	2
	Jolicoeur, Jeanne	Psychiatric Aide	2
	Jones, Florence	Psychiatric Aide	7
	Jorgens, Rosa	Psychiatric Aide	1
	Kalin, Florence	Psychiatric Aide	2
	Kay, Partricia	Psychiatric Aide	1
	Kohanski, Edgar	Psychiatric Aide	1
	Lalumiere, Mary	Psychiatric Aide	1
	Lamitie, Lee	Psychiatric Aide	1
	Landry, Alice	Psychiatric Aide	3
	Lavigne, Antonia	Psychiatric Aide	2
	Lavigne, _______	Psychiatric Aide	2
	Lawless, Josephine	Psychiatric Aide	3
	Lazarro, Carmen	Psychiatric Aide	½
	Lazarro, Vinc___	Psychiatric Aide	1
Nursing Service	Lee, Alexander	Psychiatric Aide	1
	Leiper, Joan	Grad. Nurse	1
	Leschinsky, Scunley	Psychiatric Aide	2
	Lillie, Elva	Psychiatric Aide	4
	Lindquist, Myr___	Charge Nurse	3
	Lunt, Burton	Psychiatric Aide	4
	Lunt, Lois	Psychiatric Aide	5
	Macomber, Henry	Psychiatric Aide	2
	Majewski, Caroline	Psychiatric Aide	1
	Marshall, Roamund	Psychiatric Aide	1
	Matassa, Maria	Psychiatric Aide	2
	Matkowski, Beatrice	Psychiatric Aide	1
	Matthews, Louise	Psychiatric Aide	2
	McCarthy, Kathleen	Charge Aide. (Psy.)	6
	MoMahon, Lucille	Psychiatric Aide	1
	Mierzejewski, Anna	ChargeAide(Psy.) (Comp.)	3

DEPARTMENT	NAME	POSITION	NO. OF DAYS
	Moran, Elsie	PsychiatricAide (Comp.)	30
	Niestzyzewski, Sophie	Psychiatric Aide	1
	Osborne, Lizzls	Psychiatric Aide	1
	Ostrowski, Mildred	Psychiatric Aide	2
	Ouellett, Raymond	Psychiatric Aide	1
	Ouimet, Martin	Psychiatric Aide	1
	Overlock, Irene	Psychiatric Aide	2
	Pasqualini, Eunice	Graduate Nurse	3
	Pavey, Florence	Psychiatric Aide	2
	Pavey, Wilbur	Psychiatric Aide	2
	Pawlak, Helen	Psychiatric Aide	1
	Perras, Robert	Psychiatric Aide	9
	Perry, Inez	Charge Aide (Psy.)	1
	Phillips, Mary	Charge Nurse	1
	Phillips, Mary	Charge Nurse (Comp.)	7
	Philpot, Esme	Psychiatric Aide	1
	Phalen, Joseph	Psychiatric Aide	13
	Phoenix, Margaret	Charge Aide (Psy.)	1
	Piechowski, Charles	Psychiatric Aide	1
	Pierce, Jay	Charge Aide (Psy.)	1
	Piezzo, Thomas	Psychiatric Aide	2
	Piontkowski, Mollie	Psychiatric Aide	4
	Pisapia, Celina	Psychiatric Aide	1
	Plante, Doris	Psychiatric Aide	2
	Preavy, Rita	Psychiatric Aide	2
	Previtera, Rose	Psychiatric Aide	1
	Reynolds, Georgianna	Psychiatric Aide	2
	Richardson, Delvina	Psychiatric Aide	1
	Rokowski, Raymond	Psychiatric Aide	1

DEPARTMENT	NAME	POSITION	NO. OF DAYS
	Rudolph, Edwin	Psychiatric Aide	1
	Rushford, Theresa	Psychiatric Aide	3
	Rydzewski, Mary	Psychiatric Aide	14
	Scofield, Annette	Psychiatric Aide	2
	Shea, Elezabeth	Psychiatric Aide (Comp.)	30
	Shea, Virginie	Psychiatric Aide	1
	Sheffield, Helen	Psychiatric Aide	1
	Smallridge, Ann	Psychiatric Aide	½
	Smith, Arthur	Psychiatric Aide	1
	Spurgas, Eillen	Graduate Nurse	1
	Sugga, Norma	Psychiatric Aide	1
Nursing Service	Suntheimer, Marie	Psychiatric Aide	2
	Talbot, Mary	Psychiatric Aide	1
	Tattoon, Eleanor	Psychiatric Aide	1
	Tellier, Theresa	Psychiatric Aide	1
	Thomas, Mertha	Charge Aide(Psy.) (Comp.)	2
	Thompson, Rose	Psychiatric Aide	½
	Tracey, Patricia	Psychiatric Aide	1
	Urban, Edith	Psychiatric Aide	2
	Vuono, Peter	Psychiatric Aide	5
	Wasik, Anne	Psychiatric Aide	1
	Watson, Doris	Psychiatric Aide	2 ½
	Watson, Doris	Psychiatric Aide (Comp.)	8
	Wehr, Rudolph	Psychiatric Aide (Comp.)	30
	Westerberg, Erlind	Psychiatric Aide	3
	Wilson, Lucia	Graduate Nurse	1
	Zaborowski, Virginia	Psychiatric Aide	4

LEAVE OF ABSENCE
JUNE 1953

DEPARTMENT	NAME	POSITION	NO. OF DAYS
Business Office	Hathaway, Lor____o	Inst. Patrolman	3
	Magowan, Georg_	Supv. Inst. Patrolman	2
	McMullan, Hel___	Tel. Operator	1
	Pershaec, Elizabeth	Typist, Gr. II	5 ½
Dietary	Goepfert, George	Inst. Helper	1
	Martin, Harold	Inst. Helper	1
Laundry	Camley, Lyle	Mgr. of Lndry. Services	½
	Aubin, Paul	Laundry Supv.	½
	Lonardelli, John	Laundry Supv.	½
	Lukaszewicz, Jeanne	Laundry Worker	½
	Minucci, Lillian	Laundry Worker	½
	Morrissette, Martin	Cleaner	2
Main Kitchen	LaPuc, Joseph	Cook	1
	Riley, John	Inst. Helper	1
	Sewart, Norman	Cook	2
	Torrance, Frederick	Head Cook	1
	Tusia, Frank	Inst. Helper	1
Maintenance	Holdorf, Fred	Steam Fireman	1
	Johnson, Walter	Chief Stat. Engineer	1
	Landry, Philip	Skld. Trdsm.	1

DEPARTMENT	NAME	POSITION	NO. OF DAYS
	Ramsay, Paul	Skld. Trdsm.	3
Medical	Ranger, Con_____ M.D.	Asst. Supt.	3
	Allan, Joseph, M.D.	Sr. Physician (Psy.)	1
	Bence, Vincent	Pharmacist	2
	Doerr, William, M.D.	Asst. Physician	1
Medical	Miller, Edward, M.D.	Resident (Psy.)	1
	Nelson, Pierce, M.D.	Asst. Physician	½
	Steinecke, Olga, M.D.	Sr. Phys. (Psy.)	2
	Zimmerman, Jervi_	Sr. Phys. (Psy.)	2
Nursing Off.	Riden, Emily	Nurse Clin. Instr.	1
	Shields, Eloise	Asst. Dir. Of Nurs. (Psy.)	2
Occup. Therap.	Kromer, Harry	Occup. Therap. Supv.	1
	Bubz, Clyde	Occup. Therapist	1
	Rosebrooks, Marjorie	Occup. Therapist	½
Prison Ward	Barton, James	Guard Attendant	3
Social Service	Capon, Joseph	Supv. Of Psy. Soc. Serv.	5
Transportation	Freeman, Arthur	Garage Foreman	½
Nursing Service	Bezovs, Lydia	Graduate Nurse	1 ½
	Blais, Walter	Psychiatric Aide	1
	Boudreau, Robert	Psychiatric Aide	1
	Bouthillier, Helen	Psychiatric Aide	1

DEPARTMENT	NAME	POSITION	NO. OF DAYS
	Callahan, Frederick	Psychiatric Aide	3
	Casler, Caroline	Charge Nurse	1
	Clay, Dorothy	Psychiatric Aide	1
	Cornish, Mary	Psychiatric Aide	1
	Cote, Francis	Psychiatric Aide	6
	Downing, Ernest	Psychiatric Aide	1
	Francoeur, Alberta	Psychiatric Aide	1
	Gagliardo, Frank	Psychiatric Aide	3
	Gagnon, Loretta	Psychiatric Aide	3
	Greenwood, Phyllis	Psychiatric Aide	1
	Gwiazdowski, John	Psychiatric Aide	1
	Hildebrand, Augusta	Charge Aide (Psy.)	1
	Jakubielski, Anthony	Psychiatric Aide	3
	Jaroch, Gale	Psychiatric Aide	3
	Jaroch, Jean	Charge Nurse	3
	John, Arlene	Charge Nurse	1
	Kalin, Florence	Psychiatric Aide	1
	Kendall, Edith	Psychiatric Aide	4
	McCoy, Genevieve	Psychiatric Aide	2
	McCready, Madeline	Psychiatric Aide	1
	Niescezewski, Lena	Psychiatric Aide	1
	Pierce, Jay	Charge Aide (Psy.)	5
	Renshaw, Margaret	Psychiatric Aide	1
	Rygielski, Ann	Psychiatric Aide	3
	Scofield, Annette	Psychiatric Aide	1
	Sewart, Marie	Psychiatric Aide	2
	Smallridge, Ann	Psychiatric Aide	½
	Tremko, Lillian	Charge Nurse	2
	Wells, Albert	Psychiatric Aide	½
	Westerberg, Erlind	Psychiatric Aide	1
	Yeznach, Elizabeth	Charge Nurse	2 ½

NORWICH STATE HOSPITAL
PERSONNEL DEPARTMENT
MONTHLY ACTIVITY REPORT
JUNE 1953

Applications		57
Rejected	17	
No vacancy	17	
Not suitable	3	
Poor references	1	
Not qualified	2	
Pending reference check	20	
Number of June applicants hired	1	
Number of June applicants hired	13	
Classifications and total number of employees hired		29
Guard Attendant	1	
Psychiatric Aide	19	
InstitutionHelper	4	
Farmhand	1	
Resident (Psy)	2	
Telephone Operator	1	
Assitant Physician	1	29
Separations		23
Transfer	1	
Left without Notice	4	
Dropped During Working Test Period	2	
Resigned	16	23

Reasons for Resignation:		
Pregnancy	4	
Better Position	3	
Illness	4	
Personal Reasons	4	
Leaving State	1	16
Student Nurse	Employed	6
Student Nurse (O.T.)	Employed	15
Student Nurse (Theology)	Employed	6
Student Nurse	Employed	34
Student Nurse (O.T.)	Separation	5
Student Nurse	Separation	21

PSYCHOLOGICAL LABORATORIES REPORT FOR JUNE 1953

Psychological services:

	Inpatients	Outpatients	Employees	Total
Interviews	--	119	--	119
Intelligence Testing	47	10	49	106
Personality Testing	53	7	--	60
Memory and Deterioration Testing	3	--	--	3
Miscellaneous Testing	5	--	--	5
Research Testing	--	--	49	49
Total	108	136	98	342

Education:

Dr. Charles P. Fonda, Senior Clinical Psychologist, lectured to the student nurses on "Psychologist, lectured to the student Nurses on "Psychological Techniques" (first session).]

REPORT OF NURSING SERVICE
JUNE 1953

On June 25, eighteen students completed the twelve weeks course in Psychiatric Nursing; on June 18 and 21, two students completed the course. Thirty-four students began their affiliation on June 16.

Nineteen aides continued in the program of theory and practices: Orientation to Psychiatric Nursing.

On June 11, a group of nurses from this hospital attended the meeting of the Catholic Nurses Organization in Greenville. Dr. Friel of our staff was the speaker.

On June 15, a group of nurses from this hospital attended a picnic of District #5, C.S.N.A. at Connecticut College for Women in New London.

On June 18, the Graduate Nurse Group of this hospital sponsored a picnic at Gardner's Lake.

Three occupational therapy students joined the nursing staff as psychiatric sides for the summer months and are assisting with our recreational program on the wards.

WARD PARTIES		
	Men	Women
Number of Parties	2	3
VISITORS TO PATIENTS		
Number of Patients Attending	272	380
Number of Patients Visited	551	552
Number of Visitors	1566	1821

PACKAGES RECEIVED FOR PATIENTS			
Men	No. Rec'd.	Women	No. Rec'd.
Trousers, Pr.	4	Dresses	52
Top shirts	14	Slips	26
Sweater	1	Sweaters	4
Underwear, Pcs.	17	Underwear	47
Pajamas, Pr.	2	Pajamas, Pr.	1
Slippers, Pr	1	Nightgowns	5
Shoes, Pr.	1	Shoes, Pr.	19
Socks. Pr.	12	Stockings, Pr.	51
Misc. Pkgs.	113	Misc. Pkgs.	112
Food	54	Food	123

REPORT OF THE HOSPITAL BARBERS
AND BEAUTY SALON
JUNE 1953

BARBERS' REPORT	
Number of Haircuts by Barbers	696
Number of Haircuts by Patients Barbers	602
Total Haircuts	1298
Number of Shaves by Barbers	1103
Number of Shaves by Psychiatric Aides	5324
Number of Shaves by Patient Barber	391
Total Shaves	6818
Number of Self Shaves	8036
Grand Total Shaves	14854
Average Number of Shaves per Patient	10

BEAUTY SALON REPORT

	Salon Appointments	Ward Appointments
Haircut.	224	260
Shampoo	754	9
Hairset	696	9
Permanent Wave	64	1
Facial Hair Removed	45	57
Facial	11	
Eyebrow Arch	7	

Marcel	40	
Manicure	336	
Scalp Treatment	27	
Rinse	9	
Total Receiving Service in Beauty Salon	942	
Total Receiving Beauty Service on Wards	273	
Grand Total	1215	

MAINTENANCE SUMMARY REPORT
JUNE 1953

Number of Minor Repairs Complete		2309
Minor Repairs Labor Cost	$5,850.25	
Minor Repairs Material Cost	4,766.56	
	$10,616.81	
Project Labor Cost	$1,797.00	
Project Material Cost	895.43	
	$2,692.43	

POWER HOUSE REPORT

Steam Generated	17,096,200 lbs.
Oil Consumed	160,538 gals.
Evaporation	13.3 lbs.
K.W.H Generated	329,500
Average Temperature	74.8°F
Degree Days	18.1

REPORT OF THE HOSPITAL FLORIST

GREENHOUSE:	
Alyssum	1,000
Asparagus Plumosis	½ bench
Asparagus Sprengeri	½ bench
Astars	30
Carnations	625
Chrysanthemunms	1,900
Coleus	20
Ferns	12
Feverfew	200
Petunia	100
Zinnia	1,000

NURSERY:	
American Arbor Vitae	60
Catalpa	20
Elm	48
Forsythia	18
Norway Spruse	260
Douglas Fir	_1
Privet	65
Maples	125
Compacta	58
Plumosa Aurea	48
Plumosa Retina	53
Plumosa Squarossa	70

FARM REPORT
JUNE 1953

	Home Produced Vegetables
	Used During The Month
Radishes	3,540 lbs.
Lettuce	5,832 lbs.
Swise Chard	3,950 lbs.
Tur_ips	1,800 lbs.
Cabagge	300 lbs.
Asparagus	609 lbs.
Spinach	8,695 lbs.
Parsley	101 lbs.
	Purchased Vegetables Used
	During Month
Tomatoes	151 1/2 lbs.
Potatoes	64, 200 lbs.
Cauliflower	47 heads
String Beans	108 ½ lbs.
Onions	4,180 lbs.
Lettuce	2,263 heads
Cucumbers	96 lbs.
Celery	3,144 bunches
Carrots	4,174 lbs.
Cabbage	11,525 lbs.
Egg Plant	52 lbs.
Sweet Potatoes	140 lbs.

NORWICH STATE HOSPITAL
NORWICH, CONN.

Financial Statement for month of June 1953

"A" Personal Service Appropriation			$	3,252,391.00
	Committed to July 1, 1953	$	141,251.27	
	Expended to July 1, 1953		3,111,139.73	3,252,391.00
	Balance			$ 0.00
"B" Contractual Service Appropriation			$	242,950.00
	Committed to July 1, 1953	$	33,947.28	
	Expended to July 1, 1953		208,995.18	242,942.46
	Balance			$ 7.54
"C" Supplies & Materials Appropriation			$	
	Committed to July 1, 1953	$	44,011.05	1,206,782.00
	Expended to July 1, 1953		1,146,824.79	1,190,835.84
	Balance			$ 15,946.16
"J" Equipment Appropriation (two year account)			$	64,061.09
	Committed to July 1, 1953	$	3,452.89	
	Expended to July 1, 1953		60,565.11	$ 64,018.00
	Balance			43.09

"Q" Structural Changes-Major Improvements				$	59,281.43
	Committed to July 1, 1953	$	1,938.93		
	Expended to July 1, 1953		49,253.41		51,192.34
	Balance			$	8,089.00
"H" New Structures				$	48,756.80
	Committed to July 1, 1953	$	6,094.93		
	Expended to July 1, 1953		30,047.12		36,142.05
	Balance			$	12,614.75
Bond Issue				$	2,771,066.49
	Committed to July 1, 1953	$	1,702,026.16		
	Expended to July 1, 1953		786,761.68		2,488,787.84
	Balance			$	282,278.65

NORWICH STATE HOSPITAL
PER CAPITA COST PER PATIENT

Based on Storeroom Issues for July 1953

94	Total Patient Days		Employees Meals	24,109			
3145.1	Patient Average Days		Employees & Families	5,820			
			Total	29,929			
			Avg. Day (3 meals)	332.5			
						PER CAPITA COST	
							Inc. Emp.
		Value	Month	Week		Day	Per Day
General Groceries	$	26,447.30	8.409	1.962		0.280	0.254
Milk & Cream		9,471.29	3.011	0.703		0.100	0.090
Fresh Fruits & Vegs.		7,252.46	2.306	0.538		0.077	0.069
Meat		13,920.46	4.426	1.033		0.147	0.133
Fish		10,116.78	0.323	0.075		0.011	0.01
FOOD TOTAL	$	58,108.29	18.475	4.311		0.615	0.556
Bedding	$	1,244.12	0.396	0.092		0.013	

Cleaning		1,540.16	0.49	0.114	0.016
Household, Misc.		3,227.39	1.026	0.239	0.034
Office		385.05	0.122	0.029	0.004
Tobacco & Cigarettes		885.99	0.282	0.066	0.009
Yard Goods		2,410.32	0.766	0.179	0.025
Men's Clothing		3,633.10	2.465	0.575	0.082
Women's Clothing		3,722.42	2.225	0.519	0.076
Misc. Total	$	17,048.55	7.772	1.813	0.259
Grand Total	$	75,`56.81	26.247	6.124	0.874

NORWICH STATE HOSPITAL
JUNE 28–JULY 4, 1953

BREAKFAST MENU, AS SERVED

SUNDAY		
CONGREGATE	EMPLOYEES	STAFF
Stewed Prunes, Puffed Wheat	Fresh Oranges, Puffed Rice	Pineapple Juice, Cold Cereal
_umb Coffee Cake	Soft Cooked Eggs, Crumb Coffee	Bacon & Eggs any Style
___ite Bread, Margarine	Cake, White Bread, Toast	White, Hye Bread, Toast
Coffee	Margarine—Coffee	Muffins, Grape Jelly, Margarine
MONDAY		
Oranges, Farina	Tomato Juice, Puffed Wheat or	Chilled Tomato Juice, Maltex
__iddle Cakes & Syrup (Men)	Farina w/ Milk, Scrambled Eggs	Cold Cereal, Bacon & Eggs
__eamed Eggs (Women)	White Bread, Toast, Margarine	any style, White, Dark Bread
White Bread, Margarine	Marmalade	Toast, Margarine, Grape Jelly
Coffee	Coffee	Coffee, Milk
TUESDAY		
Stewed Prunes, Wheatena	Stewed Prunes, Puffed Wheat or	Chilled apricots, Wheatena
__eamed Eggs (Men)	Wheatena w/Milk, Fried Eggs	Cold Cereal, Eggs any Style
Pancakes & Syrup (Women)	Sugared Doughnuts, White Bread	Grilled Bacon, White, Rye Bread

White Dark Bread, Margarine	Toast, Margarine, Jelly	Toast, Margarine, Plum Jelly
Coffee	Coffee	Coffee, Milk
WEDNESDAY		
Tomato Juice, Puffed Rice w/Milk	Fresh Oranges, Puffed Wheat	Stowed Prunes, Farina, Cold
Doughnuts, White Bread	French Toast & Maple Syrup	Cereal, Eggs any style, Grille
Margarine	White Bread, Toast, margarine	Bacon, Sugar Doughnuts, Toast
Coffee	Coffee	White Bread, Margarine
		Apple Jelly— Coffee, Milk
THURSDAY		
Oranges, Wheatena	Orange & Grapefruit Juice	Sliced Banana w/ cream, Maltex
French Toast & Syrup (Men)	Puffed Wheat or Wheatena w/Milk	Cold Cereal, Eggs any style
Soft Cooked Eggs (Women)	Bacon & Eggs, White Bread	Grilled Bacon, White Bread
White & Dark Bread, Margarine	Toast, Margarine, Jelly	Toast, Margarine, Apple Jelly
Coffee	Coffee	Coffee, Milk
FRIDAY		
Tomato Juice, Oatmeal	Stewed Prunes, Puffed wheat or	Stewed Prunes, Farina, Cold
Soft Cooked Eggs (Men)	Oatmeal w/Milk, Plain or O__let	Cereal, Bacon & Eggs any style
French Toast & Syrup (Women)	White Bread, Toast, Margarine	White, Rye Bread, Toast
White Bread, Margarine	Jelly	Margarine, Apple Jelly
Coffee	Coffee	Coffee, Milk
SATURDAY		
Stewed Prunes, Maltex	Pineapple Juice, Puffed Wheat	Tomato Juice, Wheatena, Cold

cornbread	or Maltex w/Milk, Poached Eggs	Cereal, Eggs any style, Grill
White Bread, __ Jam	White Bread, Toast Muffins	Bacon, White Bread, Toast
Coffee	Margarine or Jam	Margarine, Apple Jelly
	Coffee	Coffee, Milk

SUPPER MENU, AS SERVED

SUNDAY		
CONGREGATE	EMPLOYEES	STAFF
__anish Rice, Cucumber Salad	Vienna Loaf, Brown Gravy, Potato	Ham Caroline on Corn Bread
Lettuce, White Bread	Puffs, Sliced Cucumbers, Diced	Baked Potato, Sliced Tomato on
Margarine, Stewed Pears	Carrots, White Bread, Margarine	Lettuce, Pickles & Olives
Milk	Canned Pears, Hot or Iced Coffee	White Bread, Margarine
		Baked Custard, Iced or Hot Coffee
		Tea, Milk
MONDAY		
Baked Macaroni & Cheese	Veal Fricassee, Sliced Beets	Chilled Fruit Cup, Corned Beef
Pickled Beets, White Bread	Buttered Rice, Sliced Cucumbers	Hash, Poached Eggs, Buttered Beet
Margarine, Oranges	White Bread, Margarine, Baked	Lettuce Salad, White Bread
Milk	Apple w/Nutmeg Sauce	Margarine, Raisin Rice Cream
	Hot or Iced Coffee	Iced or Hot Coffee, Tea, Milk
TUESDAY		
__amed Dried Beef on Toast	Creamed Dried Beef, Baked Potato	Grilled lamb Chops w/ Gravy, Squad
Freah Green Beans	Buttered Peas, Corn on the Cob	Boiled Potatoes, Corn, Lettuce
White Bread, Margarine	Garden Salad, White Bread	Salad, White Bread, Margarine
__atine w/Custard Sauce	Margarine, Oranges	Lemon Cake Pudding w/cream
Chocolate Milk	Iced or Hot Coffee	Iced or Hot Coffee, Tea, Milk

	WEDNESDAY	
___y Bean Soup, Croutons	Pea Soup, Crackers, Sliced Veal	Grilled Hamburg & Onions, French
___iced Cucumbers, Sliced	Loaf, Potato Salad on Lettuce Leaves	Fries, Buttered Corn, Carrot
Cheese, Lettuce Salad w/	Sliced Cucumbers, White Bread	Raisin Salad, White Bread, Margarine
_____sian Dressing, Dark Bread	Margarine, Marble Cake	Deep dish apple pie
Margarine, Marble Cake	Iced or Hot Coffee	Iced or Hot Coffee, Tea, Milk
	THURSDAY	
______ced Veal Loaf	Corned Beef, Hash, Fresh Green Beans	Baked Ham w/sauce, Candied Yams
_____sh String Beans, Oven	Corn on the Cob, Sliced Tomatoes	Squash, Lettuce Salad, White Bread
___n Potatoes, White Bread	Pickles, White Bread, Margarine	Margarine, Chilled Fruit
__ter, Pineapple Whip	Blanc Mange—Iced or Hot Coffee	Iced or Hot Coffee, Tea, Milk
	FRIDAY	
_____ish Cakes, Tomato Sauce	Salmon Loaf or Hamburger, Parsley	Baked Fish w/Lemon of Cheese
__tuce-Celery & Cucumber	Sauce, Cottage Fried Potatoes	Dreams, Baked Potato, Buttered
___ad, Corn on the Cob	Corn on the Cob, Sliced Tomatoes	Carrots, Lettuce Salad, White
_____ Bread, Margarine	White Bread, Margarine, Ice Cream	Bread, Margarine
_____ Cream—Milk	Iced or Hot Coffee	Old Fashion Spice Cake w/icing
		Iced or Hot Coffee, Tea, Milk
	SATURDAY	
_____ Hash w/Brown Sauce	Cream of Celery Soup, Crackers	Vaal ala King on Toast, Baked
_____ered Squash, Green Pepper	Western Omelet, French Fries	Potato, Buttered Peas, Lettuce &
___d, White Bread	Baked Summer Squash, White Bread	Tomato Salad, White Bread

Margarine, Raisin Cake	Margarine, Raisin Cake	Margarine, Bread Pudding,
	Iced or Hot Coffee	Iced or Hot Coffee, Tea, Milk

__ TE SUPPER MENU, AS SERVED JULY 20–AUG 1ST, 1953 NORWICH STATE HOSPITAL

SUNDAY
EMPLOYEES
Pot Roast of Beef, Gravy, Whipped Potatoes
Buttered peas, Corn on Cob, White Bread
Margarine, California Cream
Iced or Hot Coffee, Milk
MONDAY
Vegetables Soup, Crackers, Sliced Corn Beef
Mashed Potatoes, Fresh Swiss Chard, __ustard
Corn on Cob, White Bread, Margarine
Ice Cream—Iced or Hot Coffee, Milk
TUESDAY
Hamburg Steak, Gravy, Oven Brown Potatoes
Buttered Wax Beans, Sliced Cucumber
White Bread, Rolls Margarine
Peach Short Cake w/Custard Sauce
Iced or Hot Coffee, Milk
WEDNESDAY
Sliced Boiled Ham, Escalloped Potatoes
Boiled Cabbage Wedges, Corn on Cob

White Bread, Margarine, Mustard
Ice cream—Iced or Hot Coffee, Milk
THURSDAY
Minute Steak, Gravy, Fren_________
Fries, Fresh Summer Squash, White Bread
Lettuce Wedges w/Cream Dressing
Grapenut Custard, Margarine
Iced or Hot Coffee, Milk
FRIDAY
Corn Bisque, Crackers, Fried Fillet of Sole
or Beef Goulash, Tomato Sauce
Whipped Potato, Fresh Spinach
White Bread, Margarine, ______ Squares
Iced or Hot Coffee, Milk
SATURDAY
Baked Pork & Beans, Grill a Frankf_____t_rs
Sliced Cucumbers, Corn on Cob
Potato Salad, on lettuce, White Bread
Margarine, Pineapple Whip
Iced or Hot Coffee, Milk

NORWICH STATE HOSPITAL
___ MENU, AS SERVED

CONGREGATE	EMPLOYEES	STAFF
	SUNDAY	
_Steak, Whipped Potatoes	Roast Veal, Gravy, Franconian	Tomato Juice, Stuffed Cabbage
_nach, White Bread, Butter	Potatoes, Carrots ala King	w/Sauce, Oven Browned Potatoes
Chocolate Pudding	Lettuce Salad, White Bread	Buttered Peas & Carrots
	Margarine, Creamy Rice Pudding	Mixed Salad, White Bread, Marg.
	Iced or Hot Coffee, Milk	Pineapple Upside Down cake w/
		Whipped Cream
		Iced or Hot Coffee, Tea, Milk
	MONDAY	
_____lled Frankfurters	Swiss Steak, Gravy, Mashed Potato	Grapefruit Juice, Grilled
___anconian Potatoes, Harvard	Buttered Wax Beans, Combination	Minute Steak, French Fries
__ts, Dark Bread, Butter	Salad, White Bread, Margarine	Buttered Green Peas, Mixed Sal.
_amed Pudding	Bavarian Cream	White Bread, Margarine
Iced Tea	Iced or Hot Coffee, Milk	Gingerbread w/cream
		Iced or Hot Coffee, Tea, Milk

	TUESDAY	
__t Loaf, Gravy	Vegetables Bisque, Crackers	Chilled Tomato Juice, Assorted
___tered Rice, Diced Carrots	Fried Liver, Gravy, Whipped Potato	Cold Cuts, Potato Salad, Olives
_k Bread, Butter	Succotash, Lettuce Wedge w/Dressing	Pickles, White Bread, Margarine
Cream, Iced Tea	White Bread, Margarine	Strawberry Ice Cream
	Strawberry Cello	Iced or Hot Coffee, Tea, Milk
	Iced or Hot Coffee, Milk	
	WEDNESDAY	
_____ed Corned Beef, Buttered	Celery Soup,___ cutons, Sliced	Cream of celery Soup, Rib Roast
Potatoes, Fresh Swiss Chard	Corned Beef, Escalloped Potatoes	of Beef, Gravy, Oven _____
__uce Leaves, White Bread	Fresh Swiss Chazd, Lettuce Salad	Roasted Potatoes, Buttered
__ter, Bread Custard w/Nutmag	White Bread, Margarine, Mustard	Wax Beans, Tossed Salad
__uce—Iced Tea	Chocolate Pudding w/ sauce	Hot Dinner Rolls, Crackers
	Iced or Hot Coffee, Milk	Margarine, Apple Pie w/Cheese
		Iced or Hot Coffee, Tea, Milk
	THURSDAY	
___ed Liver, Gravy, Mashed	Sliced Boiled Ham, Baby Beets	Corned Beef, Cabbage & Carrots
Potatoes, 10 Minute Cabbage	Pickles, Potato Salad w/Egg Garnish	Boiled Potato, Mixed Salad
White Bread, Butter	Mustard, White Bread, Margarine	White Bread, Margarine

__ Cream—Iced Tea	Ice Cream—Iced or Hot Coffee, Milk	Fudge Ripple Ice Cream
		Iced or Hot Coffee, Tea, Milk
	FRIDAY	
____d Fillet of Sole	Fried Fillet of Sole or Heat Loaf	Cream of Tomato Soup, Fried
___lloped Potatoes, Buttered	Gravy, Tartar Sauce, Au Gratin	Fillet of Sole, Tartar Sauce
___rots, Lettuce & Celery Salad	Potatoes, Butter rod Spinach	Pot Roast of Beef, Whipped
White Bread, Butter	Lettuce & Celery Salad, White Bread	Potatoes, Cole Slaw, Fresh
__in Rice Pudding—Milk	Margarine, Peach Delight	Green Beans, White Bread
	Iced or Hot Coffee, Milk	Margarine, Crackers, Sour ____
		Iced or Hot Coffee, Tea, Milk
	SATURDAY	
_____cad Cold Boiled Ham	Pot Roast, Gravy, Mashed Potato	Italian Spaghetti, Meat Balls
___table Sticks, macaroni	Buttered Green Beans, White _____	Fresh Green Beans, Tossed __
______d on Lettuce, White Bread	Margarine, Ice Cream	White Bread, Margarine, ______
____, Ice Cream	Iced or Hot Coffee, Milk	Ice Cream
____ Tea		Iced or Hot Coffee, Tea, Milk

NORWICH STATE HOSPITAL
JUNE 28–JULY 4TH, 1953
__ PER MENU, AS SERVED

	SUNDAY	
CONGREGATE	EMPLOYEES	STAFF STAFF
_____atable Rice Soup, Croutons	Scotch Broth, _______, Assorted	Club Sandwich, Potato Salad
___tuce Salad w/ cream Dressing	Cold Cuts, Macaroni Salad on	Pickles & Olives, White Bread
__te Bread, Margarine	Lettuce, Relish, Mustard	Margarine, Fruited Gelatine w/
_____lesauce—Milk	White Bread, Margarine, Fruit Cup	Sauce, Iced or Hot Coffee, Tea, Milk
	Iced or Hot Coffee	
	MONDAY	
__ghetti Creole	Western Omelet, Buttered _____	Veal Chop Suey, Steamed Rice
____sed Green Salad	White Bread, Margarine, Catsup	Noodles, Green beans
__te Bread, Margarine	Lemon Cake	Pineapple & Pearsalad
____on Cake—Milk	Iced or Hot Coffee	White bread, margarine
		Chocolate Cupcakes
		Iced or Hot Coffee, Tea, Milk
	TUESDAY	

___ced Cold Cuts, Potato Salad	Beef Goulash, Buttered Noodles	Pineapple Juice, meat Balls w/
Lettuce, White bread, Butter	Diced Beets, White Bread	Gravy, Whipped Potatoes
_____sh Fruit—Milk	Margarine, Ice Cream	Cream Corn, Garden Salad
	Iced or Hot Coffee	White Bread, Margarine
		White Cake
		Iced or Hot Coffee, Tea, Milk
	WEDNESDAY	
__nish Rice, Lettuce Wedges	Hamburg Steaks, French Fries	Ragout of Beef, Buttered Peas
__ressing, White Bread	Lettuce & Tomato Salad, White Bread	Whipped Potatoes, Molded Sal.
__nut Butter, Fruit Whip	Margarine, Canned Pears	White Bread, Margarine
___________	Iced or Hot Coffee	Glorified Rice Pudding
		Iced or Hot Coffee, Tea, Milk
	THURSDAY	
__st Beef, Hash, Brown Sauce	Stuffed Cabbage, Tomato Sauce	Steamed Frankfurters, Potato
__bination Salad	Baked Potatoes, Lettuce Wedges w/	Salad, Tossed Salad, Pickles
__k Bread, Butter	Dressing, White Bread, Margarine	Olives, White Bread, Margarine
__it Squares—Milk	Fruit Squares—Iced ___ Hot Coffee	Raisin Cake—Coffee, Tea, Milk
	Friday	

__ed Fish Cakes, Tomato Sauce	Corn Chowder, Crackers, Salmon	Salmon Salad on Lettuce or
__tered Green Beans	Salad or Sliced Cold Meat	Macaroni Salad, Lettuce Wedges
__ Bread, Butter	Julienne Potatoes, Shredded	White Bread, Swiss Chard
___ Butter Cookies	Lettuce w/Dressing, Mustard	Margarine, Sponge Cake w/Icing
___	White Bread, Margarine, Peanut	Iced or Hot Coffee, Tea, Milk
	Butter Cookies-Hot or Iced Coffee	
	SATUDAY	
___ed Pork & Beans	Baked Pork & Beans, Grilled Frank-	Grilled Ham Steaks, Baked
__bage Slaw, White Bread	furters, Cabbage-Pineapple Salad	Pineapple Slices, Whipped
Margarine, Watermelon	Mustard, Relish, White Bread	Potato, Buttered Peas
	Margarine, Watermelon	Cucumber & Tomato Slices
	Iced or Hot Coffee	White Bread, Margarine
		Ice Cream on Watermelon
		Iced or Hot Coffee, Tea, Milk

NORWICH STATE HOSPITAL
JUNE 28TH,–JULY 4TH. 1953
_ SUPPER MENU, AS SERVED

SUNDAY
EMPLOYEES
Roast Veal, Gravy, Framonian Potatoes
Carrots ala King, Lettuse Salad
White Bread, Margarine
Creamy Rice Pudding
Iced or Hot Coffee, Milk
MONDAY
Swiss Steak, Gravy, Mashed Potatoes
Buttered Wax Beans, Combination Salad
White Bread, Margarine
Bavarian Cream
Iced or Hot Coffee, Milk
TUESDAY
Veg. Bisque, Crackers, Fried Liver
Gravy, Whipped Potatoes, Succotash
Lettuce Wedge w/Dressing, White Bread
Margarine, Strawberry Jello
Iced or Hot Coffee, Milk
WEDNESDAY
Celery Soup, Croutons, Sliced Corned Beef
Escalloped Potatoes, Fresh, Swiss Chard

Lettuce Salad, White Bread, Dinner Rolls
Margarine, Munt___, Chocolate Pudding
Iced or Hot Coffee, Milk
THURSDAY
Sliced Boiled Ham, Baby Peets
Potato Salad, w/Egg Garnish, Mustard, Pickles
White Bread, Magarine, Ice Cream
Iced or Hot Coffee, Milk
FRIDAY
Tomato Juice, Fried Fish or Meat Loaf
Gravy, Au Gratin Potatoes, Tartar Sauce
Butter Spinach, Lettuce & Celery Salad
White Bread, Margarine, Peach Delight
Iced or Hot Coffee, Milk
SATURDAY
___ ___, Gravy, Mashed Potatoes
Buttered Wax Beans,____ ____
Margarine, ___ ___
Iced or Hot Coffee, Milk

STATISTICAL REPORT FOR MONTH OF JULY 1953

	MEN	WOMEN	TOTAL
Movement of Population June 30, 1953	1474	1673	3147
Admitted During month by commitment	56	48	104
By Emergency	48	35	83
By Probate	4	9	13
By Secsion 2668	2	3	5
By Transfer	1	1	2
By Drug Addict	1	0	1
From extended visit	8	11	19
From temporary visit	77	180	257
From elopement	3	0	3

DISCHARGED DURING MONTH

	MEN	WOMEN	TOTAL
Discharged from hospital	22	11	33
Discharged from Emergency:	14		
Not Insane	7	1	8
Recovered	2	2	4
Unimproved	1	1	2
On extended visit	15	14	29
On temporary visit	86	199	285
Died	18	6	24
Eloped	2	0	2
Number remaining July 31, 1953	1474	1683	3157

DISCHARGED FROM HOSPITAL
RECORDS DURING MONTH

Discharged from Visit	11	17	28
From Movement	0	0	0
Changed from temporary to extended visit	2	1	3
Number out of Hospital on visit	177	218	395
On elopement	2	1	3

MOVEMENT OF POPULATION
ADMITTED DURING JULY 1952

Admitted	56	43	99
Discharged	16	4	20
Died	5	10	15
Visit	17	11	28
Family Care	1	0	1
Number remaining July 31, 1953	17	18	35

AGES OF ADMISSIONS

9_ Under	0	0	0
10-16	0	1	1
___ –29	0	0	0
__–___	5	4	9
___ ___	9	11	2_
__–___	_1	5	16
50–59	15	10	25
60–69	4	7	11
70-Over	12	10	22
_______	0	0	0
______	56	48	104
______	53._	52.55	

ACTIVITY REPORT OF THE ACUTE MEDICAL AND SURGICAL SERVICE (LIPPITT), INFIRMARIES (KIRKBRIDE, GALT, RAY, AND SEYMOUR 2), AND TUBERCULAR SERVICE (SEYMOUR 1, 3, 4).
JULY 1953

	Lippit		Ray	Kirkbride	Galt 1	Seymour 1	Seymour 2	Seymour 3	Seymour 4
	Men	Women	Women	Men	Men	Inact. TB Men	Intirmary Women	Active TB Men	Active TB Women
_at End of Previous Month	47	37	238	237	53	30	41	39	27
Admitted to Ward	29	24	6	18	6	5	2	2	3
Discharged: a. Improved	31	16	0	1	1	–	–	–	–
b. Unimproved	0	0	2	2	7	0	3	4	1
c. Death	4	0	3	10	0	1	0	0	0

SPECIAL THERAPEUTIC PROCEDURES
JULY 1953

	Men	Women	Total
	Men	Women	Total
Shock Therapy:			
Electric-convulsive	54	74	125
Insulin Shock	24	35	59
Combined EST and Insulin	0	7	7
Anti-luetic Therapy:			
Penicillin	1	1	2
Endocrine Therapy:			
Regular Insulin	2	13	15
Insulin N.P.H	1	2	3
P.Z.I.	4	20	24
Thyroid	0	1	1
Parenteral Vitamins:			
Ensolbec C	14	6	20
Betaxin	1	3	4
Liver	0	1	1
Ferrocal	0	1	1
Hypobeta	4	0	4
Special Chemotherapy:			
Penicillin	105	55	160
Sulfathiassole	0	4	4
Streptomycin	39	22	61
Gantrisin	2	0	2
Cortisone	1	2	3
Aureomycin	1	-	1

	Men	Women	Total
Terramycin	2	57	59
I.N.A.H.	1	2	3
P. A. S.	33	18	51
Special Psychotherapy:			
Individual Psychotherapy—Number of Hours	533	496	1,029
Number of Patients	132	269	401
Narcotherapy:			
Sodium Amytal Interviews	2	4	6
Physiotherapy:			
Diathermy	17	11	28
Other Applications of Heat	20	19	39
Massage	15	16	31
Passive and Corrective Exercises	67	32	99
Employees: Total No. Treatments	66	48	114
Hydrotherapy (whirlpool)	21	5	26
Vaccinations and Inoculations:			
Typhoid	39	0	39
Small Pox	28	0	28
Hydrotherapy:			
Continuous Tub			
Number of Patients	16	17	33
Number of Hours	921 ¼	452- ¾	1374
Wet Sheet Pack—			
Number of Patients	30	147	177
Number of Hours	500 ½	207 ½	2572
Number of Packs	170	688	858
Special Protective and Supportive Procedures:			
Intravenous Feedings	0	8	8
Clyses	20	8	28

	Men	Women	Total
Blood Transfusions	0	11	11
Restraints:			
Sheets	3	58	61
Mittens	0	9	9
Wrists	12	1	13
Wrists and Anklets	2	0	2
Camisole	1	0	1
Total Number of Hours	708	10795 ½	11503 ½
Seclusion:			
Number of Patients	30	90	120
Number of Hours	2270	13,442	15,712
TOTAL NUMBER OF PATIENTS RECEIVING TREATMENTS	797	1,077	1,874

SPECIAL DIAGNOSTIC PROCEDURES
JULY 1953

	Men	Women	Total
Lumber Puncture	7	2	9
EEG	20	15	35
EKG	43	40	83
BMR	1	1	2
Gastric Lavage			85

HYDROTHERAPY REPORT
JULY 1953

	Men	Women	Total
WET SHEET PACKS:			
	170	688	858
Number of Packs	500 ½	2071 ½	2,572
Number of Hours	30	147	177
Number of Patients			
RESTRAINTS:			
Number of Camisole	1	0	0
Number of Wrists and Ankles	2	0	2
Number of Wrists	12	1	13
Number of Mittens	0	9	9
Number of Sheets	3	58	61
Humber of Hours (total)	708	10795 ½	11503 ½
Total Number of Patients	18	68	86
SECLUSION:			
Number of Patients	30	90	120
Number of Hours	2,270	13,442	15,712
HYDROTHERAPY (CONTINUOUS TUB):			
Number of Patients	16	17	33
Number of Hours	921 ½	452- ¾	1,374

PHYSICIANS' MONTHLY REPORT
JULY 1953

A. Medical—Surgical Clinic (Employees)	Men	Women	Total
Number of Employees Treated	71	116	187
Hospitalized	3	7	10
Number of Hospital Days	38	30	68
Physical Examinations on New Employees	8	12	20
Physical Re-examination (food and milk handlers)	8	6	14
Compensation Forms	12	32	44
Typhoid Immunization	14	10	24
	116	183	299
B. Medical—Surgical Outpatient Clinic (Patients)	Men	Women	Total
Number of Patients—Surgical	17	19	36
Number of Patients—Medical	18	26	44
Gyn. Examinations	0	10	10
	35	55	90
C. Consultations—Visiting Staff	Men	Women	Total
Eye (nonclinic cases)	9	6	15
Ear, Nose, and Throat (nonclinic cases)	1	0	1
Surgery	4	4	8
	14	10	24
Chiropody	51	80	131
	65	90	155

SPECIAL SUMMARY ENTERIC SERVICES
JULY 1953

Number of Typhoid Carriers 6 (women)

SPECIAL PSYCHIATRIC EXAMINATION AND DIAGNOSTIC
PROCEDURES (PSYCHIATRIC)
JULY 1953

	Men	Women	Total
Routine Weekly Psychiatric Review Notes	203	185	388
Rountine Monthly Psychiatric Review Notes	131	160	291
Routine Semi-Annual Psychiatric Review Notes	13	13	26
Routine Annual Psychiatric Review Notes	99	108	207
Admission Mental Status Examinations	56	48	104
Letters Answered Reviewing Psychiatric Condition	72	59	131
Number Cases Presented to General Staff Conference	3	2	5
Number Cases Presented for Consideration of Release	39	35	74

SURGICAL REPORT
JULY 1953

	Number of Operations		
Major Surgical Procedures:	Men	Women	Total
Herniorrhaphy, left	1	-	1
Lobotomy, Standard	1	1	2
Pinning of Hip, right	-	2	2
Supracondylar Leg Amputation, right	2	-	2
Right Temporal Lobe Tumor, Bilateral burr	-	1	1
	4	4	8
Minor Surgical Procedures:	Men	Women	Total
Amputation of finger, right hand	-	1	1
Bronchoscopy	2	-	1
Biopsy, right breast	-	1	1
Debridement	5	4	9
D. And C. Of Uterus	-	1	1
Incision and Drainage of Infection	4	7	11
Liver Biopsy	-	1	1
Lumbar Puncture	1	1	2
Luetic Lumbar Puncture	4	-	4
Removal of Fingernail	1	1	2
Removal of Foreign Body	2	-	2
Repair of Lacerations	5	2	7
Pnuemoperitoneum	1	-	1
	25	19	43

Fracture Treatment:	Men	Women	Total
Fracture Olecranon. Plaster Cast	1	-	1
	1	0	1

REPORT OF THE _____ ____
JULY 1953

Type of Test	Number of Tests
Urinalysis:	
Routine	435
Sugars	269
Acetone	31
Bile	2
Urobilinogen	1
Diacetic Acid	1
Culture	1
Glucose Tolerance	2
Hematology:	
Hemoglobin	308
W. B. C.	300
R. B. C.	308
Differential	308
Sedimentation Kate	23
Typhoid	11
R. H. Factor	6
Cross-matching	11
Pyothrobin Time	1
Hematocrit	6
M. C. Volume	1
M. C. Volume Concentration	1
M.C. Hemoglobin	1
Chemistry:	
Urea Nitrogen	198
Sugar	271
Creatinine	38

Type of Test	Number of Tests
N. P. N.	24
Total Protein	4
Albumin	4
Globulin	4
Icteric Index	1
Bilirubin	1
Alk. Phosphatase	2
Cholesterol	3
Cephalin Flocculation	5
Chlorides	1
Stools:	
Culture	
Occult Blood	227
Bile	4
	2
T. B. Culture:	
Culture	123
Smears	5
Serology:	
V. D. R. L	124
Kolmer	10
Spinals:	
Kolmer	31
Pandy's	21
Cell Count	31
Protein	26
Smears	22
Chloride	3
Sugar	5
Culture	6
Colloidal Gold Curve	30
Special Tests:	
Vaginal Smear	1
Throat Culture	2

Type of Test	Number of Tests
Tooth Culture	32
Total Number of Laboratory Tests	3268
Histology Slides	326

REPORT OF AUTOPSIES AND DEATHS
JULY 1953

	Men	Women	Total	
Number of Deaths	18	6	24	
Number of Autopsies	8	2	10	41 %
Number of Medico-Legal Cases	4	2	6	

CAUSES OF DEATH AS SHOWN ON AUTOPSY REPORTS

1. Jack Heller—male

Anatomical Diagnosis: Generalized Arteriosclerosis; Hypertrophy and dilatationof the left ventricle of the heart; Fibrosis of the Myocardium; Syphilitic aortitis; Left hydrothorax; Edema of the right lung; Old healed pleurisy; Suppurative bronchitis; Senile arteriosclerotic kidneys; Hypertrophy of the Prostate; Ascites; Chronic passive congestion of the viscera

Clinical Diagnosis" Acute cardiac dilatation; Syphilitic heart disease; General Paresis

2. Alex Rachewski—male

Anatomical Diagnosis: Generalized arteriosclerosis; Dilatation of the ventricles of the heart; Fatty infiltration of the myocardium; Bilateral apical pulmonary tuberculosis; Hypertrophy of the prostate; Chronic passive congestion of the viscera

Clinical Diagnosis: Acute Cardiac Dilatation; Arteriosclerotic heart disease

3. Charles Robertson—male
Anatomical Diagnosis: Carcinoma of the lung with metastasis to the paricardium, mediastinum, pleurae, bronchial lymph glands, diaphragm and liver; Generalized arteriosclerosis; Hypertrophy and dilatation of the ventricles of the heart; Fibrosis of the myocardium; Right hydrothorax, Old healed pleurisy (left side); Edema of left lung; Bilateral bronchopneumonia; Ascites; Senile arteriosclerotic kidney; Cyst of left kidney; Hypertrophy of the prostate

Clinical Diagnosis: Cancer of Liver with metastases; Arteriosclerotic heart disease; Generalized Arteriosclerosis

4. Anthony Philips—male
Anatomical Diagnosis: Generalized arteriosclerosis; Hypertropy and dilatation of the ventricles of the heart; Acute peritonitis; Ascites; Incarcerated right hernia; right __ healed pleurisy; Left hydrothorax; Emphysema (right upper lobe); Bronchopneumonia and suppurative bronchitis (left lower lobe); Cholelethiasis (infective stone) _____ arteriosclerosis kidney; Cystic kidney; Chronic passive congestion of viscera

Clinical Diagnosis: Cancer of Liver with metastases; Arteriosclarotic heart disease; Generalized Arteriosclerosis

5. James Costello—male
Anatomical Diagnosis: Generalized arteriosclerosis; Obliterating pericarditis; dilatation of the ventricles of the heart; Fibrosis and fatty infiltration of the myocardium; Suppurative bronchitis; Fibrino-purulent pleurisy; Bronchopneumonia kidney; Hypertrophy of the prostate; Right strangulated hernia Myxoma of the left thigh; Chronic passive congestion of the viscera

Clinical Diagnosis: Bronchopneumonia; Generalized arteriosclerosis; Intestinal obstruction

6. Harry Boughton—male
Anatomical Diagnosis: Generalized arteriosclerosis; Bilateral bronchopneumonia (lower lobes); Suppurative Bronchitis; Old healed pleurisy; Senile arteriosclerotic kidneys; Hypertrophy of the prostate

Clinical Diagnosis: Arteriosclerosis heart disease; Generalized arteriosclerosis; Bilateral suppurative bronchopneumonia

7. Anne Grant—female
Anatomical Diagnosis: Generalized arteriosclerosis; Hypertrophy and dilatation of the ventricles of the heart; Fibrosis of the myocardium; Old healed pleurisy; Bronchopneumonia (right lung) Suppurative bronchitis;

Senile artariosclerotic kidney; Fibroma and polyp of the uterus; Chronic passive congestion of the viscera

Clinical Diagnosis: Bilateral bronchopneumonia; Generalized arteriosclerosis; Hypertensive Cardiovascular disease

8. George Lamelle—male
Anatomical Diagnosis: Generalized arteriosclerosis; Hyper-trophy and dilatation of the ventricles of the heart; Fibrosis of the myocardium; Old healed pleurisy (left side); Suppurative bronchitis; Carcinoma gelatinosum of the rectum with multiple metastases to both lungs and the bronchial lymph glands; Moderate cirrhosis of the liver; Senile arteriosclerotic kidneys; Multiple abscesses of the kidney; chronic passive congestion of the viscera

Clinical Diagnosis: Cerebrovascular accident; Generalized and advanced Arteriosclerosis; Carcinoma of Rectum with Pulmonary metstases

9. Frank J. Scheblein—male
Anatomical Diagnosis: Generalized arteriosclerosis; Fibrosis of the myocardium; Bilateral old healed pleurisy; Congestion of the left lung (lower lobe); Senile arteriosclerotic kidney

Clinical Diagnosis: Generalized arteriosclerosis; Respiratory center failure; Senile psychosis

    10. Ellen Bowler—female

Anatomical Diagnosis: Generalized arteriosclerosis; Hypertrophy and dilatation of the ventricles of the heart; Mitrak stenosis; Aortic stenosis and insufficiency; Fibrosis of the myocardium; Lobar pneumonia (right lower lobe); Senile arteriosclerotic kidneys; Anus preternaturalis (artificail arms); Colostomy. Peritonitis; Gangrene of the small intestine; Missing rectum and sex organs; Chronic passive congestion of the viscera

Clinical Diagnosis: Acute intestinal obstruction with gangrene; Old abdominal perineal resection of Rectum with adhesions, for Adenocarcinoma; Acute cardiac dilatation with arteriosclerotic heart disease; Fracture, right ilian; Senile psychosis

CAUSES OF DEATH AS GIVEN ON DEATH CERTIFICATES AND AGES AT DEATH

	Age at Death
1. Bronchopneumonia; Advanced Rheumatoid Arthritis	58
1. Acute cardiac Dilatation; Syphilitic Heart Disease	62
1. Arteriosclerotic Heart Disease; Generalized Arteriosclerosis	65
1. Acute Cardiac Dilatation; Arteriosclerotic Heart Disease	65
1. Lobar Pneumonia (left); Left Hydrothorax; Art. Ht. Disease	78
1. Cancer of Liver with Metastases; Art. Ht. Disease	87
1. Arteriosclerotic Heart Disease; Generalized Arteriosclerosis	87
1. Sarcoma of Stomach; Arteriosclerotic Heart Disease	76
1. Arteriosclerotic Heart Disease; Generalized Arteriosclerosis	90
1. Recurrent Pneumonia; Art; Ht. Disease; Gen. Arteriosclerosis	74
1. Bronchopneumonia; Myocarditis; Arteriosclerosis	83
1. Bronchopneumonia; Arteriosclerotic Heart Disease	73
1. Myocardial Failures; Arteriosclerotic heart disease	93
1. Bronchopneumonia; Generalized Arteriosclerotic' Intestinal Obstruction	83
1. Arteriossclerotic Heart Disease; Generalized arteriosclerosis	62
1. Rheumatic Carditis with Mitral Stenosis; Subacute Endocarditis	39
1. Bilateral bronchopneumonia; Generalized arteriosclerosis	76

1.	Bronchopneumonia; Art. Ht. Disease	73
1.	Carebrovascular accident; Gen. And Adv. Arteriosclerosis; Ca. of rectum with Pulmonary Matastasis	85
1.	Status Epilepticus; Chronic Alcoholism	44
1.	Generalized arteriosclerosis; Bronchopneumonia; Intratrochanteric Fracture, right femur	74
1.	Generalized arteriosclerosis; Respiratory Center Failure	81
1.	Acute Intestinal Obstruction with Gangrene; Old Abdominal Perineal Resection of Rectum with adhesions	81
1.	One patient ___ at the Stratford _______ Home, 7/24	
Average Age at Death		74

REPORT OF THE HOSPITAL
X-RAY DEPRATMENT
JULY 1953

Part Examined	Examinations		Films
Abdomen	6		6
Ankle	11		17
Arm	15		17
Chest	259		265
Cholecystogram	1		4
Femur	2		2
Foot	9		10
G. I. Series, Stomach and Fluoroscopy	6		18
G. I. Series, Colon and Fluoroscopy	2		6
Hand	18		20
Hip, Routine	13		30
Hip, Pinning	2		20
Jaw	1		4
Knee	5		6
Leg	7		8
Mastoids	2		11
Nose	3		7
Pelvis	18		19
Ribs	9		21
Shoulder	13		27
Skull, Routine	23		87
Spine, Cervical	1		3
Spine, Dorsal	59		64
Spine, Lumbar	10		21
Spine, Sacrum and Coccyx	4		11
Wrist	7		7
Trachea	1		3

Part Examined	Examinations		Films
Total:	507		714
Number of Patients Examined		401	
Superficial Therapy Treatments		2	

Part Examined	Examinations		Films
Total:	507		714
Number of Patients Examined		401	

SOCIAL SERVICE REPORT
JULY 31, 1953

CASE COUNT

Extended Visit	Male	Female	Total
Carried Over	167	203	370
Added During Month	17	15	32
Total	184	218	402
Closed			
Discharge of Patient	11	17	28
Return of Patient	8	11	19
Closed during month	19	28	47
CARRIED FORWARD	165	190	355
Family Care (Regular)			
Carried Over	9	9	
Added During Month	2	1	
Total	11	10	
Closed			
Extended Visit Granted		1	1
Return of Patient		1	1
Total	0	2	2
CARRIED FORWARD	11	8	19
Family Care (Dr. Friedman's Conval. Home)			
Carried Over	20	15	35
Added During Month			

Total	20	15	35
Closed			
Return of Patient			
Discharged			
Deceased			
Total	0	0	0
CARRIED FORWARD	20	15	35
Family Care (Golden Heights Chronic and Convalescent Hospital)			
Carried Over	6	19	25
Added During Month	0	0	0
Total	6	19	25
Closed			
Extended Visit Granted or Disch.	0	0	0
Return of patient	0	0	0
Deceased	0	0	0
CARRIED FORWARD	6	19	25

SOCIAL SERVICE REPORT

Family Care (Stratford Chronic and Convalescent Hospital)	Male	Female	Total
Carried Over	25	14	39
Added During Month	3	0	3
Total	28	14	42
Closed			
Extended Visit or Discharged			
Return of Patient	1	1	2
Deceased		1	1
Total	1	2	3
CARRIED FORWARD	27	12	43
GRAND TOTAL IN FAMILY CARE CONVALES. HOMES	53	46	99
Pre-Visit Studies			
Carried Over	3	8	11
Added During Month			
Total	3	8	11
Closed			
Visit Granted	1		1
Visit Refused			
Total	1		1
CARRIED FORWARD	2	8	10
Number of Interviews for			
Supervision of patient on visit			8
Supervision of patient in Family Care			57

Pending Placement of patient in Family Care			4
Family Care Home Finding			
Psychiatric Social Histories			49
Pre-Visit Studies			14
Personal Services			25
Total			157

	Total	Grand Total
3. Person Interviewed		
Patient	84	
Relative	63	
Collateral	10	
Total		157
4. Place of Interview		
Hospital	129	
Field	28	
Total		157
5. Hartford Clinic Interviews (Social Worker)		
Periodic Routine Check-ups		
Patient	15	
Relative	11	
Collateral		
Psychiatric Socail Histories		
Relative		
Collateral	1	
Treatment		
Patient	2	
Relative	2	
Collateral	3	
Consultations		
Patient	2	
Relative	2	
Collateral		
TOTAL		38

HARTFORD CLINIC	OUT-PATIENT SERVICE			MONTH ENDING	July 31,1953
Caseload—Follow-up					Total
Cases carried over					135
Added during month					25
Total					160
Closed during month					15
Carried end of month					145
Caseload—Treatment					
Cases carried over					17
Added during month					1
Total					18
Closed during month					2
Carried end of month					16
Reason for Closure		Condition			
	Unimp	Imp	Much Imp	Rec'd	Total
Hospitalized	4				4
Discharged		2	9	1	12
Transferred to Follow-up		1			1
					17
Source of Referral					

Routine Follow-up	26				
Purpose of Interview		Person Seen			
	Pt.	Rel.	Collat.		Total
Follow-Up					
Check-up	43	21			64
Consultation	10	3			13
Total	53	24			77
Treatment	18	10			28
Pre-visit Contacts					
Consultation		4			4
Total Interviews	71	38			109
Conference with Other Agencies		2			
Psychological Tests					
Appointments Made					
Kept	83				
Not kept but responded	14				
Not kept—no response	17				
	114				
Telephone Calls	12				

Backus Hospital Clinic Report omitted For Month of July. See August report, Which will include July.

REPORT OF THE HOSPITAL DENTIST
JULY 1953

Procedure	Treatments	Patients
Dentures Repaired	3	3
Dentures Marked and Cleaned	53	37
Impression for Dentures	0	0
Artificail Dentures	2	1
Examinations	126	126
Extractions:		
Novocaine	37	24
N 20	0	0
Sodium Pentothol (on Lippitt)	3	1
Root-Canal Therapy	6	1
X-rays:		
Intra-oral	29	10
Extra-oral	0	0
Fillings	11	5
Prophylaxes	1	1
Treatments	17	14
Surgery:		
Surgical Extractions	2	2
Total Number of Treatments	290	
Total Number of Patients Receiving Treatment		225

OCCUPATIONAL THERAPY REPORT
JULY 1953

MEN'S ADMISSION SERVICE	
OCCUPATIONAL THERAPY SHOP	Average Daily Attendance 20
Plywood board for Chinese checkers	1
Drawer partitions	2
Refinished windsor rocker	1
Office desk (2 locks)	1
Knotted rugs (new)	2
Ash trays, copper	2

OCCUPATIONAL THERAPY REPORT
JULY 1953

WOMEN'S ADMISSION SERVICE	
OCCUPATIONAL THERAPY SHOP	Average Daily Attendance 34
Woven Rug	1
Woven Scarf	1
Table Mats	13
Potholders	11
Bed Socks, pair	2
Crochet Cotton Shawl	1
Dresser Scarves	9

OCCUPATIONAL THERAPY REPORT
JULY 1953

MEN'S OCCUPATIONAL THERAPY SHOP	Average Daily Attendance 34
Basket; drug, repaired, varnished	1
Bench; large, lawn, repainted	1
Benches; small, lawn, repaired, repainted	10
Boxes; egg, painted, labelled	4
Box; file, covered, constructed, varnished	1
Box; file, open, constructed, varnished	1
Cabinets; bedside, painted	2
Cabinet; closed, constructed, painted	1
Cabinet; open, constructed, varnished	1
Cans, low, painted	4
Can; step-on, repainted	1
Chair; commode, painted	1
Chair; commode, varnished	1
Chairs; lawn, constructed	18
Chairs; lawn, painted	4
Chairs; metal, repainted	25
Chair; metal and wood, painted	1
Chairs; plain, ward, refinished	12
Chairs; plain, ward, repainted	18
Chairs; straight, painted	2
Clothes dryers; large, folding, constructed	2
Desk; constructed, shellacked, varnished	1
Frame for hooked mats; constructed, varnished	1
Mats; chair, hooked	12
Mats; table, hooked	2
Rack; mop, constructed, painted	1
Rocker; metal, repainted	1
Rockers; porch, back and seat caned, all refinished	8

MEN'S OCCUPATIONAL THERAPY SHOP	Average Daily Attendance 34
Rocker; porch, back caned, all painted	1
Rocker; porch, seat caned, all refinished	2
Rocker; porch, new parts, varnished	1
Rug; braid weave	1
Rug; knotted	2
Rugs; woven	2
Scarves; woven	7
Signs; lettered, painted or varnished	25
Standard for Bulletin Board; repaired, varnished	1
Stand; bedside, painted	1
Stools; barber, constructed, shellacked, varnished	10
Tray; medication, constructed, shellacked, varnished	1
Tray; thermometer, constructed, shellacked, varnished	1
Wastebaskets; painted, decorated	26
Runners; woven	6

OCCUPATIONAL THERAPY REPORT
JULY 1953

SEWING ROOM		Average Daily Attendance 69	
		NEW ARTICLES	
Aprons, cafeteria, 15"			6
Aprons, cafeteria, 30"			24
Aprons, kitchen, bib style			114
Bags, laundry, small			150
Bags, laundry, large			156
Bags, disposal			24
Bed-pan covers			23
Caps, cooks', sizes 7, 7 ¼, 7 ½			96
Covers, mattress, rubber			21
Covers, mattress, 36" infirmary			14
Covers, mattress, 32" infirmary			12
Dresses, print			95
Dresses, hercutex, swirl			33
Gowns, night, women's			42
Gowns, nurses			15
Gowns, johnnie-coats			62
Harnesses			24
Pajamas, women's, pairs			28
Pajamas, men's, pairs			36
Pants, altered			39
Slips			312
Uniforms, altered			4
	TOTAL		1330

MENDED ARTICLES			
Aprons	7	Floor pads	9
Bags, canteen	1	Gowns, johnnie coats	494
Bags, laundry	20	Gowns, night	5
Bathrobes	129	Gowns, surgical	2
Ned Jackets	19	Harnesses	5
Bedsides	2	Overalls	1342
Bedspreads	37	Pajamas	1
Belts, safety	1	Pants	567
Blankets	35	Pants, cafeteria	46
Blouses, strong	25	Pillow cases	20
Cases, gloves	14	Scarf, bureau	2
Cases, pillow	1	Sheets	538
Cases, syringe	66	Sheets, hydro	18
Chair backs	9	Shirts, top	112
Coats, suit	4	Shirts, baseball	4
Covers, bedpan	2	Shorts	1
Covers, burlap	10	Slacks	53
Covers, hydro	8	Slips	14
Coveralls	17	Sweaters	18
Dresses, hercutex	4	Underwear	3
Dresses, print	16	Uniforms, red/white	24
Dresses, swirl	70	Uniforms, white	2
Flags	3	Vest	1
		TOTAL	3781

OCCUPATIONAL THERAPY REPORT
JULY 1953

SELL OCCUPATIONAL THERAPY SHOP	Average Daily Attendance 21
Colonial mats	1
Scarves, dresser	6
Scarves, bedside	9
Rugs, rag	1
Rugs, roving	1
Place mat, crocheted	1
Stole, knit	1
Vanity sets, stenciled	2
WOMEN'S OCCUPATIONAL THERAPY SHOP	Average Daily Attendance 27
Altar Cloth, hemstitched	1
Church Napkins, hemstitched	6
Curtains, pairs, made	102
Curtains Tiebacks, pairs, made	6
Dish Towels, hemmed	200
Dresser Scarves, embroidered and edges crocheted	49
Hand Towels, hemmed	272
Mouth Gags, made	1547
Night Table Scarves, embroidered and edges crocheted	11
Pockets on Jackets	10
Sseat Covers, lines	14
Shower Caps, made	6
Stockings, pairs, mended	488
Table Cloths, hemmed	36
Tea Aprons, made	50

Wash Cloths, hemmed	280
BRYAN OCCUPATIONAL THERAPY SHOP	Average Daily Attendance 48
Socks, pairs, mended	700
Dresses, mended	140
Ear Tabs	1200
Towels, hemmed	125
Laundry Tags	150
Rug Strips	
Yarn, wound	

OCCUPATIONAL THERAPY REPORT
JULY 1953

UPHOLSTERY SHOP	Average Daily Attendance 8
Chairs, refinished	5
Mattresses, constructed	31
Shades, window, repaired	30
Table, refinished	1
Venetian Blinds, repaired	4
SHOE SHOP	Average Daily Attendance 7
Belts, repaired	1
Clocks, repaired	1
Shoes, pairs, exchanged	18
Shoes, pairs, repaired half soles	20
Shoes, pairs, heeled, composition leather	23
Shoes, pairs, heeled, rubber	26
Shoes, pairs, heel linings	16
Shoes, pairs, heel pads	12
Shoes, pairs, insoles	1
Shoes, pairs, piece soles	31
Shoes, pairs, plates	1
Shoes, pairs, toes tipped	1
Shoes, pairs, patch and sew	31
Slippers, bed, resew soles	1
Pocketbook, repaired	1
MEN'S OCCUPATIONAL THERAPY	
PRINT SHOP	
Pads Glued	512

Pads Glued (Used paper)	319
Triple Holes Punched (Multigraph Impressions)	500
Assembled and Stapled (Duplicating Impressions)	1708
Double Holes Punch (Multigraph Impressions)	9892
Manifold	3000
Duplicating Impressions	18026
Printing Impressions	19972
Multigraph Impressions	26260

OCCUPATIONAL THERAPY REPORT
JULY 1953

OCCUPATIONAL THERAPY MENDING ROOM SELL BUILDING	Average Daily Attendance 29
Apron	1
Bathrobes	24
Blouses	45
Blouses, strong	3
Coveralls	1
Dresses	3681
Gowns, night	441
Gowns, nurses	45
Pajama coats	69
Pajama pants	114
Pants	8
Shirts, top	919
Shorts	354
Skirts	23
Slacks, farmerette	4
Slips	1110
Underwear, female	739
Union suits	236
Underdrawers	2
Undershirts	205

OCCUPATIONAL THERAPY REPORT
JULY 1953

RECREATIONAL THERAPY REPORT	No. Times	Av. Attendance
Classes in Roller Skating	50	34
Soft Ball Games	14	87
Lawn Games	52	43
Club House Activities		
Bell	4	38
Dix	1	10
Mitchell	4	25
Woodward	2	6
Brigham	4	28
Stribling	1	20
Gallup	4	28
Moving Pictures (Wards)		
Seymour 3	3	39
Seymour 1	3	34
White	2	100
Galt	2	57
Kirkbride 3	2	54
Kirkbride 1	2	90
Gallup 2	3	44
Salmon 2	3	32
Salmon 1	3	42
Lippitt	2	10
Seymour 2	3	42
Seymour 4	3	27
Ray 3	2	90
Dix	2	45
Bell 1	2	53
Mitchell 1	2	20
Lippitt 4	2	20

Cutter	2	120
Bryan	1	125

July 4—the Norwich Women of the Moose sponsored the 4th of July entertainment for 1211 patients who were able to attend the outdoor festivities. The program consisted of variety of numbers, such as ballet, tap, acrobatic, toe, Irish and Spanish dances, vocal and accordian solos and numbers by a kitchen band which was composed of the women of the Moose. Following the entertainment, refreshments were served by Occupational Therapy students under the direction of the Occupational Therapy Department.

July 14—seventy-four veterans attended a party given at the Club House by the Norwich and Old Lyme units of the American Legion Auxiliary. Several quiz programs, group singing and dancing were enjoyed and delicious refreshments were served.

	No. Times	Av. Attendance
Bingo Parties		
Salmon I	5	
Salmon II	5	
Stribling I	4	
Stribling II	4	
White	4	
Earle	4	
MUSIC THERAPY REPORT		
Choir Rehearsals	8	24
Group Singing (Ray O.T. Shop)	3	

OCCUPATIONAL THERAPY REPORT
JULY 1953

RELIGIOUS SERVICES

Catholic Services July 5, 12, 19, 26 (Theatre)
Protestant Services July 5, 12, 19, 26 (Theatre)
Protestant Services on wards: Bryan, Ray 2, Ray 3, Kirkbride 1, Kirkbride 3, Seymour 2, Seymour 3, Seymour 4, and Salmon 1 & 2 on alternate Sundays

OCCUPATIONAL THERAPY
WARD PROJECTS

Lippitt 3	2" x 2" gauze compresses, doz.	223
	4" x 4" gauze compresses, doz.	918 ½
	ABD pads	1591
Lippitt 4	2" x 2" gauze compresses, doz.	666
Stribling	Chairs, sanded	20
	Beds, sanded	10
	Bedside stands, sanded	4

OCCUPATIONAL THERAPY REPORT
JULY 1953

On July 1, four patients from the Men's Admission Service attended the matinee performance of *"Gentlemen Prefer Blondes"* at the Norwich Summer Theatre. They were accompanied by an employee.

On July 8, four patients from the Women's Continued Treatment Service (Woodward and Awl), accompanied by an employee, attentded the matinee performance of *"The Postman Always Rings Twice"*, starring Barbara Payton and Tom Neal at the Norwich Summer Theatre.

On July 15, four patients from the Galt Building, accompanied by an employee, attended the Norwich Summer Theatre to see the play "Bell, Book and Candle", starring Alexis Smith and Victor Jory.

On July 22, four patients from Dix 2, accompanied by an employee, saw the play, *"Mister Roberts"* at the Norwich Summer Theatre.

Four patients from the Earle Building, accompanied by an employee, attended the Norwich Summer Theatre where they saw the matinee performance of *"Personal Appearance"*, starring Dagmar.

The tickets to these performances were made available to our patients through the courtesy of the Norwich College Club and Mr. Herbert Kneeter, manager of the Norwich Summer Theatre.

OCCUPATIONAL THERAPY REPORT
JULY 1953

NORWICH STATE HOSPITAL
WOMEN'S AUXILIARY

On July 6, members of the Women's Auxiliary, Mrs. Brambilla, Mrs. Sandberg, Mrs. Lynch, and Mrs. Stoudtvisited patients in the Seymour Building.

On July 23, Mrs. Lowech, Mrs. Osten, Mrs. Peele, and Mrs. Dixon visited patients in the Bryan Building.

OCCUPATIONAL THERAPY REPORT
JULY 1953

On July 13, Miss Marie Louise Franciscus, O.T.R., Director of Training Courses at the Columbia University, visited the Occupational Therapy Department and interviewed affiliating Occupational Therapy students from that University.

On July 14, Mr. Harry Kromer, O.T.R., Director of Occupational Therapy, attended a meeting of the Advisory Committee on Standards for Textiles of the State Purchasing Department in Hartford.

On July 15, Miss Nancie B. Greenman, O.T.R., Associate Professor of Occupational Therapy and Miss Patricia Laurencellem O.T.R., Assistant Director of

Occupational Therapy at the University of Kansas, visited the Occupational Therapy Department and interviewed affiliating students from the University of Kansas.

OCCUPATIONAL THERAPY REPORT
JULY 1953

REPORT ON INDUSTRY	Average Daily Attendance
Main Kitchen	35
Dining Room, Congregate	41
Dining Room, Employees	6
Laundry	36
Engineering Department	13
Housekeeping	57
Store Room	5
Farm and Barns	63
Others	322
	————————
	578
Ward Work	330
Ward Classes	31

OCCUPATIONAL THERAPY REPORT
REPORT OF THE GENERAL LIBRARY
JULY 1, 1953–AUGUST 1, 1953

TOTAL CIRCULATION 3236
TOTAL ATTENDANCE 1181

CIRCULATION IN THE LIBRARY:	
Books issued to patients	372
Books issued to employees	8
Magazines issued	851
Newspapers issued	221
Puzzles issued	89
CIRCULATION ON WARDS:	
Books issued	75
Magazines distributed	1489
Newspapers distributed	104
Puzzles distributed	27
READING ROOM ATTENDANCE:	
Ward Groups	77
General Attendance	1104
MAGAZINES RECEIVED:	
Subscriptions	24
No. received on subscription	30
No. gift magazines	1893
BOOKS RECEIVED:	
Gifts	104
Purchased	none

ACCOUNTING REPORT:	
No. books catalogued	4282
No. new books added	26
No. books lost/destroyed	10
No. books in Patients Library	4266
No. books in Seymour Library	487
No. book in Mitchell Library	79
No. books in Gallup Library	124
No. books in Bell Library	157
No. books in Bryan Library	44
TOTAL NUMBER OF BOOKS:	5173

MEDICAL LIBRARY
MONTHLY REPORT
JULY 1953

Number of books in library		4128
Number of books added		3
Total number of books in library		4131
Number of books circulated		359
Number of journals subscribed to		90
Number of journals received		93
Number of journals circulated		111
Interlibrary Loans		3
Material from MLA Exchange		7
Books added		
Quarterly Cumulative Index Medicus, vol. 50		
Hackett—Carboard Giants		
Gift—The Nephrotic Sydrome		
	JULY CIRCULATION	

Year	Books and Journals		
1950	211		
1951	304	Increase	93
1952	324	”	20
1953	470	”	146

ACCIDENT REPORT
JULY 1953

___EN	No.	Women	No.
Lippitt	1	Lippitt	3
Seymour	3	Seymour	3
Salmon	2	Awl	8
__righam	6	Bell	23
_hite	19	Cutter	15
__tribling	8	Dix	11
		Beauty Salon	1
__arle	5	Butler	10
		Sewing Room	1
__alt	8	Woodward	9
		Bryan	6
Gallup	21	Ray	28
		Stedman	5
Kirkbride	14	Mitchel	27
Total	87	Total	150

ANALYSIS OF ACCIDENTS

CAUSES OF ACCIDENTS	No Injury	Minor	Major
Cuts:			
Metal		7	
Falls:			
General	3	52	2
Convulsive Seizures		6	
Quarrels between Patients		40	
Unprovoked Attacks		41	
Self-inflicted	1	19	
Collision	1	10	

CAUSES OF ACCIDENTS	No Injury	Minor	Major
Recreational Activity		14	
Industrial Activity	1	7	
Resistiveness to Routine Care		3	
Burns		11	
Combined Irritative Treatment		1	
Undetermined		18	
	6	229	2

REPORT OF THE HOSPITAL (PROTESTANT) CHAPLAIN JULY 1953

I.		THE MINISTRY OF WORSHIP:		
	1.	Number of Worship Conducted		17
	2.	Total attendance at these 17 Services		1422
	3.	Average Attendance per Sunday (Theatre)		181
	4.	Number of Ward Services, Infirmaries and Salmon Building		13
	5.	Total Attendance at these 13 Services		697
	6.	Number of Sermons Preached		3
II.		THE SACRAMENTAL MINISTRY:		
	1.	Number of Holy Communion Services Conducated		1
	2.	Total Attendance at the Holy Communion Service		178
	3.	Number of Patients Receiving Holy Communion at this Service		56
III.		THE PASTORAL MINISTRY TO PATIENTS:		
	1.	Initial Religiou Interviews with Newly Admitted Patients		1
	2.	Number of Patients on Danger List visited		23
IV.		HOSPITAL TEACHING CLINICAL PASTORAL TRAINING:		
	1.	Number of Students in Training		7
	2.	Chaplain's Conferences with Resident		18
			Hours:	25
	3.	Chaplain's Conferences with Other Students		21
			Hours:	34

	4.	Resident's Conferences with Other Students		14
			Hours:	30
	5.	Seminars Led by Chaplain		16
			Hours:	29
	6.	Seminars Led by Resident		7
			Hours:	11
	7.	Grand Total Hours in Formal Teaching Activities		120

PUBLIC RELATIONS
JULY 1953

VISITORS TO HOSPITAL	
July 28, 1953.	Mr. John C. Leith, newly appointed Director of Nursing at the Connecticut State Hospital at Middletown, accompanied by three members of his staff, visited the hospital and spent the day seeing the wards and discussing mutual problems of administration and education.
July 30, 1953.	Mr. Philip A. Johnson and Mr. Philip I. Howay of the Hospital Board spent the morning at the Hospital visiting several patient buildings and making a tour of the grounds.

MEETINGS ATTENDED	
July 8, 1953.	Dr. Ronald _____ attended a meeting of the hospital superintendents at the Hotel Bond, Hartford.
July 9, 1953.	the Annual Meeting of the Board of Trustees was held at the summerhouse of the chairman. Mrs. G. Gardiner Russell on Buffalo Bay, Madison, Mr. Boynick of the Joint Committee of State Mental Hospitals, and Doctor Kettle, the hospital superintendent, were present. The officers of the board for the coming year are:
	Mr. Philip A. Johnson, President
	Mr. Lawrence A. Vineburgh, Vice President
	Mrs. Edwin W. Higgins, Secretary
July 9, 1953.	Mr. Zimmerman and Mr. Melican, Social Service workers, attended a meeting of the United Workers in Norwich.

July 9, 1953.	Dr. George Duffes, physician in charge of outpatient services, accompanied by Sidney Orgel, clinical psychologist, attended a meeting of the United Workers in Norwich. They participated in a discussion concerning the hospital's outpatient services.
July 14, 1953.	Mr. Harry Kromer, Director of Occupational Therapy, attended a meeting of the Advisory Committee on Standards for Textiles of the State Purchasing Department in Hartford.
July 16, 1953.	Dr. Kettle attended a meeting of the Chronically Ill, Aged, and Infirm at the Office of the Joint Committee in Hartford.

Examining Board (Personnel)
Dr. Kettle was one of the examiners on the Committee for appointment of a Chief of Medicine for the Chronically Ill, Aged, and Infirm.

PUBLIC RELATIONS REPORTED BY HOSPITAL CHAPLAIN
Addresses Related to Chaplain's Work: 7/10/53. Morning Devotions, Radio Station WICB 7/17/53. Morning Devotions, Radio Station WICB
One address was by the Resident Chaplains, Mr. Carpenter, the other by the Hospital Chaplain, Mr. Zimmerman.

(HOSPITAL CHAPLAIN) (assisted in community churches)
Reverend Zimmerman assisted in the services at Christ in Norwich on July 5, 19, at 8:00 a.m., and on July 5 and 26 at 11:00 a.m.

Sermons Preached in Community Churches
The chaplain was the guest preacher at Christ Church in Norwich on July 12 and at the United Congregational Church in Norwich on July 19. He also conducted the services on those dates.

Professional Meetings Attended	
July 7.	the Chaplain met with the Committee on Ministry in Public Institutions on this date. The meeting was in Hartford.
July 23.	the hospital chaplain and all Students held their Midsummer conference of clinical pastoral training at the Norwich State Hospital.

23 EMPLOYEES ENTERED THE SERVICE DURING JULY 1953

NAME	POSITION	DATE
Elinor Wozniak	Institution Helper	7/1/53
Charlotte Capallo	Telephone Operator	7/1/53
Gary Morris, M. D.	Asst. Physician	7/4/53
Jane Morris	Charge Nurse	7/6/53
Walter Dehm, M. D.	Resident (Psy.)	7/6/53
John Hagwood	Steam Fireman	7/6/53
Virginia, Love, M. D.	Asst. Physician	7/8/53
Rosilda Czikowsky	Psy. Aide (O.T.)	7/9/53
Jennie Smith, Rein.*	Psychiatric Aide	7/9/53
Laszlo Csovanyos, M. D.	Resident (Psy.)	7/13/53
Anthony Fratoni	Institution Helper	7/15/53
Yvonne Suprenant	Institution Helper	7/20/53
Elaine O'Neill	Graduate Nurse	7/20/53
William Cimikoski	Psychiatric Aide	7/22/53
William Sharkey	Psychiatric Aide	7/22/53
Albina Grabowy	Laundry Worker	7/23/53
Charles Joseph, Jr.	Storesclerk	7/27/53
Doris Guertin	Psychiatric Aide	7/27/53
Ann Kozlowski	Institution Helper	7/27/53
Paul Lambert	Psychiatric Aide	7/28/53
Arthur Phillips	Cleaner	7/28/53
Paul Frechette	Institution Patrolman	7/29/53
Frances Gonch, Rein.*	Psychiatric Aide	7/29/53
	Former Employees—Reinstated	

21 EMPLOYEES LEFT THE SERVICE DURING JULY 1953

RET. M.	Mandatory Retirement	RES.	Resigned
DISM	Dismissal	D D	Deceased
M. L.	Military Leave	LWN	Left Without Notice
NAME	POSITION	ACTION	DATE
Mary Mack	Institution Helper	RET M	7/1/53
Theresa Hildebrand	Housekeeper	RET M	7/1/53
Elery Morse	Charge Aide (Psy.)	RET M	7/1/53
Mabel Wills	Charge Aide (Psy.)	RET M	7/1/53
Francis Cote	Psychiatric Aide	DISM	7/2/53
Norman Landry	Institution Helper	M L	7/13/53
John Hooker, M. D.	Asst. Physician	RES	7/13/53
Erlind Westerberg	Psychiatric Aide	LWN	7/13/53
Yvonne Suprenant	Institution Helper	LWN	7/20/53
Frank Chester, Jr.	Psychiatric Aide	LWN	7/21/53
Norma Schaefer	Psychiatric Aide	LWN	7/21/53
Ida Scott	Laundry Worker	RES	7/22/53
Kemit Mehlinger, M.D.	Asst. Physician	RES	7/22/53
Leo Hennigan, M.D.	Asst. Physician	RES	7/22/53 N
Elizabeth Yeznach	Charge Nurse	RES	7/22/53 N
Ann Schaeffer	Charge Nurse	RES	7/22/53 N
Leo Delorme	Lab. Techinican	M L	7/23/53 N
Doris Sebastian	Graduate Nurse	RES	7/28/53
Lorenzo Hathaway	Inst. Patrolman	RES	7/28/53
Rufus Harris	Psychiatric Aide	DD	7/28/53
Michael Misiaszek	Psychiatric Aide	RES	7/31/53

7 EMPLOYEES REASSIGNED DURING JULY 1953

NAME	POSITION FROM	POSITION TO	DATE
Ester Langseth	Charge Nurse	Nurse Supv. (Psy.)	7/1/53
Regina Whitaker	Graduate Nurse	Charge Nurse	7/1/53
Ian Brown, M. D.	Sr. Resident (Psy.)	Sr. Physician (Psy.)	7/1/53
Anita Rondeau	Graduate Nurse	Charge Nurse	7/1/53
Arthur Aldi, Jr.	Cleaner	Inst. Helper	7/1/53
Charlotte Bohara	Inst. Helper	Housekeeper	7/1/53
Vincent Bence	Pharmacist	Head Pharmacist	7/16/53

SICK TIME
JULY 1953

DEPARTMENT	NAME	POSITION	NO. OF DAYS
Business Office	Dix, Pauline	Telephone Operator	21
	Schwell, Louis	Inst. Patrolman	3
	Warner, Jane	Steno., Gr. III	2
Central Clo. Room	Conway, Anna	Clothing Caretaker	2
	Schrier, Helen	Stores Clerk	1 ½
Cong. Dining Room	Chaisson, Robert	Institution Helper	1
Dental	McCormick, Thomas	Institution Helper	24
Dietary	Chabotte, Samuel	Institution Helper	2 ½
	Goepfert, George	Institution Helper	1
	Hayes, Ruth	Din. Room Supv.	1 ½
	Iacol, Vincent	Institution Helper	2
	Moran, Grace	Din. Room Supv.	20
	sevigney, Helene	Institution Helper	1
Farm	Siragusa, Richard	Farmhand	19 ½
Housekeeping	Camley, Dorothy	Institution Helper	2
	Quinn, Katherine	Housemother	3

DEPARTMENT	NAME	POSITION	NO. OF DAYS
Laboratory	Hollis, __nn	Lab. Helper (Comp.)	31
Laundry	Camley, Lyle	Mgr. Lundry Services	½
	Aubin, Paul	Laundry Supervisor	1
	Barnes, Cleveland	Laundry Worker	½
	Emback, Arthur	Laundry Worker	1 ½
	Gauthier, Edith	Laundry Worker	½
	Gromko, Anthony	Laundry Worker	1
	Hoxsie, David	Laundry Worker	1
	Kasansky, Meriam	Laundry Worker (Comp.)	31
	Krysiak, John	Laundry Worker	1 ½
	Lane, Thomas	Laundry Worker	1
	Leone, Olga	Laundry Worker	1
	Lonardelli, John	Laundry Supervisor	1
	Lukasiewicz, Jeanne	Laundry Worker	1
	Lynch, Anna	Laundry Worker	1
	Minucci, Lillian	Laundry Worker	½
	Ponatishen, Margaret	Laundry Worker	2
	Rondeau, Rachel	Laundry Worker	1
	Zinewioe, Chester	Laundry Worker	1
Main Kitchen	Edwards, James	Institution Helper	2 ½
	Morse, Henry	Head Cook	4
	Redding, James	Cook	8
Maintenance	Bush, John	Skilled Tradesman	1
	Novakowski, Vincent	Skilled Tradesman	1
	Stewart, Kenneth	Stationary Engineer	2
	Urban, Walter	Skilled Tradesman	2

DEPARTMENT	NAME	POSITION	NO. OF DAYS
Medical	__arbone, Hubert, M.D.	Hospital Clin. Dir.	1
	__ller, __dward, M.D.	Resident (Psy.)	3
Nursing Office	Riden, Emily	Nurse Clin. Instructor	1
Occup. Therapy	Cloutier, Blanche	Therapy Aide	22
	Evert, Marjorie	Occup. Therapist (Comp.)	31
	Koscinski, Joseph	Therapy Aide	½
	Leary, Frances	Head Seamstress	1
	Lewis, Patricia	Clerk, Grade II	2
	Parker, Ethel	Therapy Aide	1
	Roberts, Virginia	Sr. Occup. Therapist	½
	Rothholz, Hazel	Library Assistant	2
Prison Ward	Looby, Maurice	Charged Guard Attendant	21
Psychology	White, Richard	Psychology Intern	2
Storeroom	Mainville, Herman	Meat Cutter	2
Nursing Service	Adams, Frances	Psychiatric Aide	1
	Ainsworth, Richard	Psychiatric Aide	1
	Angelo, Anthony	Psychiatric Aide	1
	Angelo, Mary	Clerk, Grade II	1
	Aubrey, John	Psychiatric Aide	½
	Balestracci, Alfred	Psychiatric Aide	1
	Banks, Vivian	Psychiatric Aide	1
	Beauvais, Therese	Graduate Nurse	1
	Bence, Pauline	Graduate Nurse	4
	Benson, Antoinette	Psychiatric Aide	2

DEPARTMENT	NAME	POSITION	NO. OF DAYS
	Bernal, Leslie	Psychiatric Aide	½
	Bezovs, Lydia	Graduate Nurse	3
	Blanchard, Joseph	Psychiatric Aide (Comp.)	22
	Bohara, Madeline	Psychiatric Aide	1
	Brennan, Rita	Psychiatric Aide	4
	Brogno, Caroline	Psychiatric Aide	1
	Brouillard, Mary	Psychiatric Aide	1
	Burke, Mary	Charge Aide (Psy.) (Comp.)	31
	Burns, Blanche	Psychiatric Aide	1
	Butler, Clarence	Psychiatric Aide	5
	Caplet, Lorraine	Psychiatric Aide	2
	Carlson, Barbara	Psychiatric Aide	1
	Carter, Delphinea	Psychiatric Aide (Comp.)	4 ½
	Casler, Caroline	Charge Nurse	1
	Chabot, Lucy	Psychiatric Aide	1
	Charron, Anne	Psychiatric Aide	2
	Ciccarelli, Benjamin	Psychiatric Aide (Comp.)	9
	Ciccarelli, Benjamin	Psychiatric Aide	1
	Clay, Dorothy	Psychiatric Aide	1
	Clayton, Fortunata	Psychiatric Aide	1
	Cloud, Victoria	Psychiatric Aide	1 ½
	Comstock, Ralph	Psychiatric Aide	1
	Cook, Elizabeth	Psychiatric Aide	3
	Corcoran, Nora	Psychiatric Aide	1
	Corcoran, William	Psychiatric Aide	2
	Cornwell, Joan	Psychiatric Aide	1
	Cote, Helen	Psychiatric Aide	1
	Crawford, John	Psychiatric Aide	2
	Czikowsky, Ida	Psychiatric Aide	1
	Dacy, Maude	Charge Aide (Psy.)	12
	Dabrowski, Frances	Psychiatric Aide	1

DEPARTMENT	NAME	POSITION	NO. OF DAYS
	D' Andria, Ernest	Psychiatric Aide	2
	Davis, Doris	Psychiatric Aide	1
	Dayon, Dora	Psychiatric Aide	20
	Delmonte, Katherine	Psychiatric Aide (Comp.)	31
	DeLuca, Virginia	Charge Nurse	1
	Deveau, Joseph	Psychiatric Aide	1
	Deveau, Paul	Psychiatric Aide	1
	Durand, John	Psychiatric Aide	1
	Durfee, Douglas	Psychiatric Aide (Comp.)	31
	Duthrie, Dolores	Psychiatric Aide	1
	Duthrie, Jesse	Psychiatric Aide	1
	Dyer, Josephine	Psychiatric Aide	1
	Dwinell, Nancy	Psychiatric Aide	½
	Edwards, Mary	Psychiatric Aide	1
	Enos, David	Psychiatric Aide	1
	Feldmann, Margaret	Charge Nurse	1
	Fisch, Fannie	Psychiatric Aide	2
	Fish, Marjorie	Psychiatric Aide	3
	Fitch, Estelle	Psychiatric Aide	1
	Flynn, Rose	Charge Aide (Psy.)	2
	Gardner, Stella	Psychiatric Aide	2
	Garey, Jeanne	Psychiatric Aide	1
	Garrow, Harold	Psychiatric Aide	1
	Garrow, Marion	Psychiatric Aide	2
	Garvin, Jacquelin	Psychiatric Aide	1
	Garvin, Martha	Psychiatric Aide	1
	Ghent, Thelma	Psychiatric Aide	1
	Giaconia, Anthony	Barber	4 ½
	Gionet, Norman	Psychiatric Aide	1
	Glodoski, Joseph	Psychiatric Aide	2
	Guertin, Louis	Psychiatric Aide	1
	Hart, Elaine	Graduate Nurse	1
	Havens, Irving	Charge Aide (Psy.)	2
	Herrick, Joan	Psychiatric Aide	1

DEPARTMENT	NAME	POSITION	NO. OF DAYS
	Hildebrand, Augusta	Charge Aide (Psy.)	1
	Hill, Eileen	Psychiatric Aide	1
	Inch, Adele	Charge Nurse	4
	Jacques, Robert	Charge Nurse	1
	John, Arlene	Charge Nurse	1
	Labrecque, Hazel	Psychiatric Aide	4
	Lake, Effie	Psychiatric Aide	4
	Lalumiere, ____uis	Psychiatric Aide	1
	Lalumiere, __ry	Psychiatric Aide	2
	Landry, Alice	Psychiatric Aide	2
	Lassonde, ____er	Psychiatric Aide	2
	Lassonde, Vivian	Psychiatric Aide	3
	Lavorato, Marion	Psychiatric Aide	2
	Lawson, Alexandrine	Psychiatric Aide	1
	Lazzaro, Carmela	Psychiatric Aide	1
	Leclair, Domenica	Clerk, Grade I	1
	Lemoine, Dora	Psychiatric Aide	1
	Leschinsky, Stanley	Psychiatric Aide	1
	Lindquist, Myra	Charge Nurse	14
	Loftus, Elizabeth	Psychiatric Aide	1
	Macomber, Henry	Psychiatric Aide	1
	Mansfield, Mary	Psychiatric Aide	1
	Marinello, Beatrice	Psychiatric Aide	4
	Martin, George	Psychiatric Aide	5
	Matassa, Maria	Psychiatric Aide	2
	Matkowski, Beatrice	Psychiatric Aide	1
	Matthews, Louise	Psychiatric Aide	1
	McCoy, Genevieve	Psychiatric Aide	1
	McCready, Madeline	Psychiatric Aide	1
	McGeowan, Hugh	Psychiatric Aide	1
	McGuire, Lillian	Psychiatric Aide	2
	McMahon, Lucille	Psychiatric Aide	1

DEPARTMENT	NAME	POSITION	NO. OF DAYS
	McNerney, Alfred	Psychiatric Aide (Comp.)	7
	Milligan, Elizabeth	Psychiatric Aide	1
	Misiaszek, Michael	Psychiatric Aide (Comp.)	2
	Moran, Elsie	Psychiatric Aide (Comp.)	31
	Norman, Helen	Psychiatric Aide	1
	Norville, Betty	Psychiatric Aide	10
	Ouellet, Raymond	Psychiatric Aide	2
	Panskiewicz, Madelline	Psychiatric Aide	1
	Parrish, Norma	Psychiatric Aide	1
	Pasqualini, Eunice	Graduate Nurse	11
	Penn, Virginia	Psychiatric Aide (Comp.)	3
	Peringer, Dorothy	Graduate Nurse (Comp.)	2
	Phoenix, Margaret	Charge Aide (Comp.)	3
	Planeta, Caroline	Psychiatric Aide	1
	Plante, Doris	Psychiatric Aide	2
	Proulx, Wilfred	Psychiatric Aide	1
	Renshaw, Margaret	Psychiatric Aide	1
	Richardson, Delvina	Psychiatric Aide	1
	Robillard, Blanche	Psychiatric Aide	1
	Rogalski, Edward	Psychiatric Aide	1
	Rygielski, Ann	Psychiatric Aide	1
	St. Garmain, Eleanor	Psychiatric Aide	1
	Saunders, Margerie	Psychiatric Aide	8
	Scalaro, Marguerite	Psychiatric Aide	1
	Sebastian, Doris	Graduate Nurse	1
	Sewart, Marie	Psychiatric Aide	1
	Shea, Elizabeth	Psychiatric Aide (Comp.)	1

DEPARTMENT	NAME	POSITION	NO. OF DAYS
	Sheffield, Helen	Psychiatric Aide	1
	Signorino, Gladys	Psychiatric Aide	1
	Sigrist, Nellie	Psychiatric Aide	1
	Stevens, Delora	Psychiatric Aide	1
	Suggs, Norma	Psychiatric Aide	1
	Taylor, Rose	Psychiatric Aide	1
	Tellier, Theresa	Psychiatric Aide	1
	Thomas, James	Psychiatric Aide	1
	Thomas, Martha	Charge Aide (Psy.) (Comp.)	11
	Thompson, Rose	Psychiatric Aide	5
	Trask, Elizabeth	Charge Aide (Psy.)	1
	Vanchon, Wilfred	Psychiatric Aide	1
	Watson, Doris	Psychiatric Aide	1
	Watson, Doris	Psychiatric Aide (Comp.)	3
	Wehr, Rudolph	Psychiatric Aide (Comp.)	31
	Wells, Albert	Psychiatric Aide	1
	Wenzel, Dorothy	Psychiatric Aide	2
	Wexler, Etta	Psychiatric Aide	1
	Williams, Allen	Psychiatric Aide	½
	Yerrington, Mildred	Psychiatric Aide	1

LEAVE OF ABSENCE
JULY 1953

DEPARTMENT	NAME	POSITION	NO. OF DAYS
Central Clo. Room	Smith, Norma	Laundry Worker	3
	Soboleski, Catherine	Clothing Caretaker	1 ½
Cong. Dining Room	McKeon, Gerald	Institution Helper	1 ½
Dental	Eccleston, Alice	Dental Assistant	1
Laundry	Comtois, Joseph	Laundry Worker	1
	DeForge, Ruth	Laundry Worker	½
	Emback, Arthur	Laundry Worker	1 ½
	Morrissette, Martin	Cleaner	1
	Pineault, Aline	Laundry Worker	1
Main Kitchen	Jarvis, Edgar	Institution Helper	3
Maintenance	Mansfield, Richard	Steam Fireman	1
	Page, Arthur	Skilled Tradesman	1
	Thoutte, Gerard	Skilled Tradesman	3
Medical	Taylor, Malcolm, M.D.	Hosp. Clinical Dir.	½
	Zimmerman, Jervis	Chaplain	1

DEPARTMENT	NAME	POSITION	NO. OF DAYS
Nursing Office	Shields, Eloise	Asst. Dir. Nurs. (Psy.)	17
Occup. Therapy	Kromer, Harry	Occup. Therap. Supv.	2
	Hallas, James	Psychiatric Aide	1
Personnel Office	Jervis, Marion	Personnel Officer	1
Psychology Dept.	Scales, Margaret	Clinical Psychologist	31
Nursing	Banks, Vivian	Psychiatric Aide	½
	Browne, Katrina	Psychiatric Aide	1
	Chester, Frank	Psychiatric Aide	3
	D' Andria, Ernest	Psychiatric Aide	3
	Dorsey, Barbara	Psychiatric Aide	1
	Gadue, Marie	Psychiatric Aide	½
	Grant, Barbara	Graduate Nurse	1
	Green, Clarie	Psychiatric Aide	1
	Hebert, Laurelle	Graduate Nurse	1
	Lake, Effie	Psychiatric Aide	3
	Page, Katherine	Psychiatric Aide	1
	Rushford, Theresa	Psychiatric Aide	1
	Scarr, John	Barber	½
	Schaefer, Norma	Psychiatric Aide	4
	Urban, Edith	Psychiatric Aide	1
	Westerberg, Erlind	Psychiatric Aide	6

NORWICH STATE HOSPITAL
PERSONNEL DEPARTMENT
MONTHLY ACTIVITY REPORT
JULY 1953

Applications		57
Rejected		
Not suitable	6	
No vacancy	11	
Pending reference check	24	
Refused position	2	
Pending to report for duty	2	
Number of July applications hired	12	57
Classifications and total number of employees hired		23
Telephone Operator	1	
Institution Helper	4	
Psychiatric Aide	6	
Charge Nurse	1	
Assistant Physician	2	
Psychiatric Aide (O.T.)	1	
Resident (Psy.)	2	
Institution Patrolman	1	
Graduate Nurse	1	
Steam Fireman	1	
Storesclerk	1	
Laundry Worker	1	
Cleaner	1	23

Separations		21
Mandatory Retirement	4	
Dismissal	1	
Military Leave	2	
Left without Notice	4	
Deceased	1	
Resigned	9	21
Reasons for Resignations:		
Completion of Residency	1	
To stay at Home	2	
Another Position	2	
Advice of Physician	1	
Pregnancy	1	
Looking for Better Income	1	
Appointment in Electrical Field	1	9

PSYCHOLOGICAL LABORATORIES REPORT FOR JULY 1953

Psychological services:				
	Inpatients	Outpatients	Employees	Total
Interviews	--	93	--	93
Intelligence Testing	16	4	20	40
Personality Testing	17	2	--	19
Memory and Deterioration Testing	3	--	--	3
Miscellaneous Testing	1	1	--	2
Research Testing	--	--	20	20
Total	37	100	40	177

Education

Dr. Charles _. Fonda, senior clinical psychologist, lectured to the student nurses on "Psychological Techniques" (2nd session).

REPORT OF NURSING SERVICE
JULY 1953

Thirty-four affiliate students continued in the twelve-weeks course in psychiatric nursing.

Six psychiatric aides completed the program, Orientation to Psychiatric Nursing; twenty-two entered this program, three resigned, and thirteen remain.

The graduate nurse group held its final business meeting of the year. Meetings will be resumed in September.

Two graduate nurses were added to the staff, but three resigned.

WARD PARTIES

	Men	Women
Number of Parties	1	6
Number of Patients Attending	94	295

VISITORS TO PATIENTS

Number of Patients Visited	494	614
Number of Visitors	1679	1798

PACKAGES RECEIVED FOR PATIENTS

Men	No. Rec'd.	Women	No. Rec'd.
Trousers, Pr.	18	Dresses	63
Coats	1	Coats	1
Top shirts	38	Blouses	3
Sweaters	2	Slips	27
Pajamas, Pr.	2	Pajamas, Pr.	3
Underwear, Pcs.	36	Night gowns	6
Socks, Pr.	27	Underwear	58
Shoes, Pr.	14	Shoes, Pr.	24
Misc. Pkgs.	82	Stockings, Pr.	44
Food	28	Misc. Pkgs.	71
		Food	131

REPORT OF THE HOSPITAL BARBERS AND BEAUTY SALON

JULY 1953

Barbaras' Report:				
Number of Haircuts:	by Barbers	463		
Number of Haircuts:	by Patients	547		
		1010		
Number of Shaves:	by Barbers	825		
	by Aides	5573		
	by Patients	347		
		6745		
	Total			
Number of Self Shaves		7595		
	Grand Total	14337		
Average Number of Shaves Per Patient			---	
Beauty Salon Report:				
	Beauty Salon		Ward	
	Appointments		Appointments	
Haircut	205		298	
Shampoo	740		9	
Hairset	690		9	
Permanent Have	44		1	
Facial	9			
Facial Hair Removed	49		109	

Eyebrow Arch	4			
Marcel	26			
Manicure	346			
Scalp Treatment	37			
Rinse	7			
Total Number of Patients	894		320	
Total Number of Patients Receiving Beauty Salon Service				1214

MAINTENANCE DEPARTMENT
SUMMARY
JULY 1953

Number of Minor Repairs Completed			2216
Minor Repairs	Equipment Material Cost	$4,643.34	
	Labor Cost	4602.50	
	Structural Material Cost	567.43	
	Labor Cost	582.5	
	Total	$10,395.77	
Project Labor Cost		$1,886.50	

POWER HOUSE REPORT

Steam Generated	14,558,150	lbs.
Oil Consumed	133,270	gals.
Evaporation	13.6	lbs.
K.W.H. Generated	320,600	
Average Temperature	77.2°	F
Degree Days	0	

REPORT OF THE HOSPITAL FLORIST
JULY 1953

GREENHOUSE:			
Asparagus Plumosis	½ bench	Coleus	20
Asparagus Sprengeri	½ bench	Ferns	12
Carnstions	625	Feverfew	200
Chys__themums	1900	Poinsettia	375

Nursery:	
Am. Arbor Vitae	60
Elm	48
Catalpa	20
Forsynthia	18
Norway Spruce	260
Douglas Fir	41
Plumosa Ret.	53
Privet	65
Maples	125
Compacta	58
Plumosa Aurea	48
Plumosa Squan	70

FARM REPORT
JULY 1953

	Home Produced Vegetables Used During the Month	
Lettuce	8862	lbs.
Sweet Corn	37600	lbs.
Swiss Chard	6850	lbs.
Peppers	636	lbs.
Beet	1250	lbs.
Cabbage	4060	lbs.
Tomatoes	375	lbs.
Cucumbers	4800	lbs.
Squash, summer	8000	lbs.
String Beans	7188	lbs.
Spinach	4840	lbs.
Parsley	132	lbs.
	Purchased Vegetables Used During the Month	
Tomatoes	284	lbs.
Potatoes	71200	lbs.
Cauliflower	12	heads
String Beans	52	lbs.
Onion	4725	lbs.
Lettuce	1434	heads
Cucumbers	220	lbs.
Celery	2937	bunches
Carrots	3225	lbs.
Cabbage	7950	lbs.
Egg Plant	24	ea.
Sweet Potatoes	30	lbs.

NORWICH STATE HOSPITAL
NORWICH, CONN.

Financial Statement for the month of July, 1953

"A" Personal Service Appropriation		$ 848. 578.00
Committed to Aug. 1, 1953	$ 418,698.17	
Expended to Aug. 1, 1953	138,791.83	557, 490.00
Balance		$ 291, 088.00
"B" Contractual Service Appropriation		$ 82,000.00
Committed to Aug. 1, 1953	$ 35,068.68	
Expended to Aug. 1, 1953	446.13	35,514.81
Balance		$ 46,485.19
"C" Supplies & Materials Appropriation		$ 340, 617.00
Committed to Aug. 1, 1953	$ $122,394.83	
Expended to Aug. 1, 1953	55,299.99	177,694.82
Balance		$ 162922.18
"J" Equipment Appropriation (two year account)		$ 10,000.00
Committed to Aug. 1, 1953	$ 2,502.38	
Expended to Aug. 1, 1953	1,815.15	4,317.53
Balance		$ 5682.47
"Q" Structural Changes-Major Improvements		$ **
Committed to Aug. 1, 1953	$ 1,932.38	
Expended to Aug. 1, 1953	6.35	
Balance		$
"H" New Structures		$ **
Committed to Aug. 1, 1953	$ 6,094.93	
Expended to Aug. 1, 1953		
Balance		$

Bond Issue		$ **
Committed to Aug. 1, 1953	$ 1,630,613.42	
Expended to Aug. 1, 1953	98,123.99	
Balance		$
Prepared 8/6/53		
**Pending final year-end reconciliation of Comptroller's Office.		

NORWICH STATE HOSPITAL
PER CAPITA COST PER PATIENT

Based on Storeroom Issues for August 1953

								Inc. Emp.
97,777	Total Patient Days	Employees Meals	24,984					
3154.1	Patient Average Days	Employees & Families	6,200					
		Total	31,184					
		Avg. Day (3 meals)	335.3					
		PER CAPITA COST						
		Value		Month	Week	Day	Per Day
General Groceries	$	27,582.00		8.745	1.975	.282	.255
Milk & Cream		9,700.27		3.075	.694	.099	.089
Fresh Fruits & Vegs.		9,424.19		2.987	.674	.096	.087
Meat		16,079.52		5.099	1.151	.165	.149
Fish		1,299.96		.412	.093	.013	.012
FOOD TOTAL		64,085.94		20.318	4.587	.655	.592
Bedding		1,154.36		.366	.084	.012	
Cleaning		2,058.00		.653	.147	.021	
Household, Misc.		3,910.71		1.239	.273	.039	
Office		319.99		.102	.021	.003	

Tobacco & Cigarettes		1,040.79	.329	.112	.011	
Yard Goods		1,636.44	.519	.119	.017	
Men's Clothing		3,657.83	2.482	.56	.08	
Women's Clothing		5,694.92	3.384	.763	.109	
Misc. Total		19,473.04	9.074	2.079	0.292	
Grand Total		83.558.98	29.392	6.666	0.947	

_STATE HOSPITAL
BREAKFAST MENU, AS SERVED

CONGRAGATE	SUNDAY EMPLOYEES	STAFF
___nges, Maltax, Doughnuts	Orange Juice, Puffed Rice w/ Milk	Grape Juice, Oatmeal, Cold Cereal
___ Bread, Margarine	or Maltex, Soft Cooked Eggs	Bacon & Eggs any style, Toast
Coffee	Doughnuts, White Bread, Toast	Doughnuts, White, Rye Bread
	Margarine, Jelly—Coffee	Margarine, Grape Jelly
		Coffee, Milk
	MONDAY	
__wed Peaches, Puffed	Oranges, Puffed Wheat w/ Milk	Apricots, Farina, Cold Cereal
___ w/ Milk, White Bread	Scrambled Eggs, White Bread, Toast	Bacon & Egg any style, Toast
__nch Toast & Syrup (Men)	Margarine, Marmalade	Doughnuts, White, Rye Bread
scrambled Eggs (Women)	Coffee	Margarine, Grape Jelly
___garine—Coffee		Coffee, Milk
	TUESDAY	
___efruit Juice, Wheatena	Stewed Peaches, Puffed Wheat or	Grapefruit Juice, Wheatena
scrambled Eggs (Men)	wheatena w/ Milk, Griddle Cakes	Cold cereal, Eggs any styles, Ham
__nch Toast & Syrup (Women)	& Syrup, White Bread, Toast	White, Rye Bread, Toast

____ Bread, Margarine	Margarine, Jelly	Margarine, Grape Jelly
Coffee	Coffee	Coffee, Milk
	WEDNESDAY	
__ges, Puffed Wheat w/ Milk	Tomato Juice, Puffed Wheat w/ Milk	Canned Apricots, Oatmeal, Cold
Rice w/ Applesauce	or Hot Rice w/ Applesauce, Fried	Cereal, Griddle Cakes Syrup
White Bread, Margarine	Eggs & Bacon, White Bread, Toast	Eggs any style, White, Rye Bread
Coffee	Margarine—Coffee	Grilled Bacon, Margarine, peach
		Jelly—Coffee, Milk
	THURSDAY	
__ed Stewed Fruit, Farina	Oranges, Farina or Cornflakes w/	Sliced Bananas w/ cream, Maltex
____d Eggs (Men)	Milk, Peached Eggs, Doughnuts	Cold Cereal, Eggs any style
Doughnuts (Women)	White Bread, Toast, Margarine	Grilled Bacon, Doughnuts, Toast
White Bread, Margarine	Marmalade—Coffee	White, Rye Bread, Margarine
Coffee		Peach Jelly—Coffee, Milk
	FRIDAY	
____to Juice, Oatmeal	Mixed Stewed Fruit, Oatmeal or	Stewed Prunes, Farina, Cold Cereal
Doughnuts (Men)	Cornflakes w/ Milk, French Toast	Eggs any style, Grilled Bacon
_____d Eggs (Women)	& Syrup, White Bread, Toast	Sugar Doughnuts, White, Rye Bread
Bread, Butter	Margarine, Jelly	Toast, Margarine, Peach Jelly
Coffee	Coffee	Coffee, Milk
	SATURDAY	

___wed Fruit, Maltex	Grapefruit Juice, Puffed Wheat or	Chilled Grapefruit Juice, Wheat
___ Bread, White Bread	Maltex w/ Milk, Soft Cooked Eggs	Cold Cereal, Eggs any style
Coffee	Corn Muffins, White Bread, Toast	Grilled Bacon, White, Rye Bread
	Margarine, Jam	Toast, Margarine, Peaach Jam
	Coffee	Coffee, Milk

__ STATE HOSPITAL
DINNER MENU, AS SERVED

CONGRAGATE	SUNDAY EMPLOYEES	STAFF
__ss Steak, Brown Gravy	Pot Roast of Beef, Gravy	Chilled Fruit Cup, Roast Leg of
__sley Boiled Potatoes	Whipped Potatoes, Buttered Peas	Veal, Gravy, Creamed Carrots
___tered Green Beans	Corn on Cob, White Bread	Whipped Potato, Chef's Salad
___te Bread, Butter	Margarine, California Cream	White Bread, Margarine, White ca__
__terscotch Pudding-Iced Tea	Iced or Hot Coffee, Milk	Iced or Hot Coffee, Tea, Milk
	MONDAY	
__ced Corned Beef	Vegetable Soup, Crackers, Sliced	Vegetable Soup, Roast of Beef
__pped Potatoes, Buttered	Corned Beef, Mashed Potatoes	Buttered Squash, Whipped Potatoes
__bage, Dark Bread, Butter	Fresh Swiss Chard, Corn on Cob	Cole Slaw, Brown Gravy, White Bread
_____ Cream—Iced Tea	White Bread, Margarine, Mustard	Margarine, Starwberry Ice Cream
	Ice Cream-Iced or Hot Coffee, Milk	Iced or Hot Coffee, Tea, Milk
	TUESDAY	
__t Loaf, Gravy, Mashed	Hamburg Steaks, Gravy, Oven Brown	Tomato Juice, Chicken Croquettes
Potatoes, Corn on Cob	Potatoes, Fresh Green Beans	Sauce, Buttered Green Peas

__ced Cucumbers, Pan Biscuits	Sliced Cucumbers, Rolls, White	Whipped Potato, Mixed Salad
White Bread, Jam, Rice Pudding	Bread, Margarine, Peach Short Cake	White Bread, Margarine, Pineapple
----	w/ Custard Sauce, Hot or Iced Coffee	Upside Down Cake w/ cream
	Milk	Iced or Hot Coffee, Tea, Milk
	WEDNESDAY	
__ced Boiled Ham, Mashed	Sliced Boiled Ham, Escalloped	Chicken Rice soup, Grilled Steaks
Potatoes, Fresh Swiss Chard	Potatoes, Boiled Cabbage Wedges	French Fries, Buttered Green Beans
Corn on Cob, White Bread	Corn on the Cob, White Bread	Chef's Salad, White Bread, Margarine
__ter, Ice Cream— Icced Tea	Mustard, Margarine, Ice Cream	Banana Split w/ Banana Ice Cream
	Iced or Hot Coffee, Milk	Iced or Hot Coffee, Tea, Milk
	THURSDAY	
_____t Roast of Beef, Gravy	Minute Steak, Gravy, French Fries	Fresh Mellon Balls, Roast Leg of
Buttered Rice, Summer Squash	Fresh Summer Squash, Lettuce Wedges	Lamb, Lyonnaise Potatoes
Corn on Cob, White Bread	w/ Cream Dressing, White Bread	Buttered Squash, Fresh Garden Salad
Butter, Chocolate Pudding	Margarine, Grapenut Custard	Fresh Corn, White Bread, Margarine
__ed Tea	Iced or Hot Coffee, Milk	Grapenut Raisin Pie
		Hot or Iced Coffee, Tea, Milk
	FRIDAY	
__ied Fillet of Sole	Corn Bisque, Crackers, Fried Fillet	Corn Chowder, Hamburg Steak
__calloped Potatoes, Fresh	of Sole, Tartar Sauce, Beef, Goulash	Fired Fish, Tartar Sauce, French
__inach, White Bread, Butter	Whipped Potatoes, Fresh Spinach	Fries, Fried Onions & Peppers
Pineapple Pie—Iced Tea	White Bread, Margarine, Coffee, Milk	Fresh Garden Salad, Buttered Green

	Chocolate Chiffon Pie, Hot or Iced	Beans, White Bread, Margarine
		Strawberry __pell Ice Cream
		Iced or Hot Coffee, Tea, Milk
	SATURDAY	
__illed Frankfurters, Potato	Baked Pork & Beans, Grilled Frank-	Cream of Tomato Soup, City Chicken
__lad on Lettuce, Sliced	furters, Sliced Cucumbers, Mustard	Gravy, Whipped Potato, Boiled
Cucumbers, White Bread Butter	Potato Salad w/ Eggs Garnish on	Cabbage, Mixed Salad, White Bread
__ad Custard—Iced Tea	Lettuce, White Bread, Margarine	Margarine, Banana Cream Pie
	Pineapple Whip Hot or Iced Coffee	Iced or Hot Coffee, Tea

CHALLENGE—A CALLING INTO QUESTION

Now that you have read the reports of what actually happened in 1953—over sixty-six years ago—did you expect horror stories? And yes, there were many horror stories.

When the hospital was built, there were no easy cures, or in many cases, there were no cures at all. Two world wars happened, and it took the Vietnam War for doctors to finally recognize what we now call post-traumatic stress disorder (PTSD). Patients were used for experiments, and perhaps as a result, some miracle drugs were developed. Remember, there were no cures for sexually transmitted diseases back then. Patients were shackled to prevent harming themselves and others. The list goes on and is limited only by your interpretation of the reports. In November of 1992, the doctors met some of the challenges.

I chose not to write about all the stories I have

heard out of respect for the people who were patients and are still alive (as well as the thousands of employees that worked there and would rather not speak of their experiences). Basically, the security forces were *not* armed, patients and workers were indeed injured, and I would say experiments were performed. Many of the employees were not allowed in certain areas. There was a lot of hearsay and rumors. These reports are indeed real insights into mental health issues and hopefully will help bring understanding as to why mental institutions were built in the first place.

The word *insane* means "foolish; wild." I'm probably wrong, but I believe that as children, we have all been a little foolish and wild. It took not only the parents but the whole neighborhood to be involved in the rearing of children. Teachers back then had the authority to act as a parent (within limits of course), but today, God forbid if a teacher lays a hand on a student or a parent spanks their child in front of someone. Today that is considered child abuse!

The capability of thinking outside the box of normalcy is in itself a unique concept. To me, fighting words are, "You can't do that," or "We don't have a choice." If these attitudes prevail, we would be back in the Stone Age.

The truth was that, by law, several other hospitals that were responsible for the mentally ill were closed down by the state. This occured not only here in Connecticut but also in states across America. For an extended period, patients were reintroduced back into society. Many of them remained close by to the hospital and went to a nearby city. You need to understand that these people once had shelter, a bed to sleep in, food to eat, and regular access to medical care. Some of the patients had regular jobs at the hospital as so-called trustees. With the development of what came to be known as miracle drugs, patients that were released could probably be integrated into society as long as they had medication and adhered to their dosing schedule. Almost all of their demands could be met in an area called the Franklin Square section of Norwich, which later became known as the Rose of New England. It could be said that it was perhaps one huge shopping mall.

Now Franklin Square was a place where all buses congregated and travelers were within easy walking distance to theaters, restaurants, bars, grocery stores, clothing stores, retail stores, and even the famous hotel where Abraham Lincoln spent a night in 1860, the Wauregan Hotel. There were also doctors and dentists. Buses came from other cities, and there was a train station and YMCA headquarters, which were all serving the purpose of making residents and visitors feel welcomed.

The sad thing was that these people really did not know how to seek out whatever benefits they may have been entitled to, if they had any at all. They had no place to stay, and many of them became homeless. There was no one to teacn them how to integrate into a so-called normal society and how to get a job. Social service organizations did not yet exist.

Several years earlier, there were many huge factories in the surrounding towns. Manufactures of cotton, wool, rubber, and other products decided to relocate in the Southern states where folks required less of a wage and less taxes and made more money. This, of course, caused local businesses to go into a decline, as folks could no longer afford to go out and spend money as much as they used to. After all, the newly developed automobile was expensive.

I have many pleasant memories of Norwich when I was growing up. As a teenager, I felt it was a wondrous thing that I could get on the bus or train and go nearly anywhere. I could make connections, or if I had extra money, I could rent a taxi. For someone who didn't have a car, transportation was cheap, efficient, and convenient to get around. I got to meet a lot of interesting people, saw mothers breastfeeding their babies, and inhaled cigar or pipe smoke that was almost pleasant. I loved to go to the movies and, for a quarter, I could get popcorn and a soda as well as see two movies and a cartoon that ran continuously. The theaters also provided weary travelers a cheap place to rest and take a nap.

Technology changed. Drugs (both miracle drugs and bad drugs), poor planning, and, yes, even greed and corruption, occurred. The sad thing is that the homeless were used as an excuse for grants and whatever funds that were available. These funds were carelessly spent.

The Norwich State Hospital no longer exists, but the story doesn't end here.

Wikipedia says the hospital closed in 1996, but it wasn't like someone slammed the doors and kicked everyone out. Over the years, railroad service for the population ceased to exist. As people moved away, the need for mass transit also seemed to diminish. It is ironic that with the closing of many mills, the old buildings became shelters for many of those who were displaced from the state hospital. Indifference and apathy prevailed.

Now I will tell you my story…

I joined the Navy in 1958 and soon thereafter became trained as a radar operator on a P2V-7 Neptune patrol bomber. Whenever we were not on actual patrol, pilots and crew were encouraged to train as much as possible. So on a flight from Norfolk, Virginia, to Brunswick, Maine (I was flying in the bow made of clear Plexiglas, getting a good overall bird's-eye view mostly of Long Island), when the pilot asked if I wanted to do a practice bomb run, I replied, "Yes!" I scurried up to the radar position (which was in standby). "Fired it up and then took note of where we were." I could see that we were approaching New London. I gave the pilot steering directions to begin a practice bomb run up the Thames River and guided him up to within two miles of Norwich. The pilot then turned the aircraft and announced that we could not fly over cities and apologized, but he was satisfied with the directions I'd provided him. I then rushed back into the bow and managed to take aerial photographs of the area from about five thousand feet. I still have the slides of the flight.

In 1977, I retired from the Navy and I had one heck of a time trying to get a job in this area. Basically, I was overqualified and had a difficult time, especially with the pressure of a young family to support.

When I became selectman of the Town of Sprague for two years, I met the director of the newly formed South East Area Transportation (SEAT) organization. He told me of his plans and how the government allocated millions of dollars to buy buses in preparation of the future. That was back in the '80s. Today these buses are still operating and are very seldom, if ever, filled to capacity. I had originally suggested to this gentleman that they should have bought smaller, more nimble buses (twenty passengers) to get people around more quickly and economically. This would also help folks recognize that there was now a mass transit system in place. My main concern was that the Town of Sprague was not going to be serviced by these buses, and to this day, the town is still not serviced by SEAT. Years ago, the bus came to town every twenty minutes! Prior to that, trolley cars also passed through Sprague on their way from Willimantic to Norwich, and there was train service as well.

Drivers soon complained that the big buses could not easily navigate some city streets. Routes were changed to accommodate the large buses. Perhaps because they needed an excuse (I really don't know for certain), they (the city's leaders) decided to build a huge transportation center. Ironically, this transportation center was built at the lowest elevation of the city, away from what was once the hub, Franklin Square. It seemed that a location next to a sewer plant and on top of the old dump site known as Hollyhock Island was best. The entire upper level was left without a roof, and I guess they forgot to include restrooms and a seating area for folks to wait in comfort for the next bus. The turning radius of the buses remained a problem, so they took a lane of traffic and devoted it to the turning of the buses. They actually had to tear up one section seven times in all at great expense and at the result of impeding traffic flow! It was a great example of poor planning but was quickly forgotten. The WELCOME sign for visitors disappeared.

The theaters went out of business, the big post office moved out, the YMCA (which had the only swimming pool in the city) and banks closed, and many of the small businesses that existed failed. The Buckingham home, which was willed by a former governor to the veterans, was encroached upon by the city officials, leaving the veterans one or two rooms where they could conduct their meetings. The Social Security building was moved to a location that was no longer easily accessible to almost anyone on foot. The famous Wauregan Hotel was turned into low-income housing. The Norwich Bulletin relocated to what was once a railroad terminal. Diagonal to that building stands a rusted railroad bridge, which is no longer in use. At least one or two of the existing restaurants in Franklin Square area have a big sign on their front door saying that restrooms are available to customers only, leaving no transient place to go to the bathroom.

Now there is talk of building six roundabouts (traffic circles) on a major highway (West Main Street) in Norwich! Challenges and insanity still exist.

*****

THE CHALLENGES

To be blunt, I challenge you, the reader, to visit the areas I referenced and spread the word of the astonishing ongoing transformation and miracles. See for yourselves the amazing two casinos that are considered world-class entities. You don't have to be a gambler to visit them, as in addition to gambling there are numerous restaurants, high-end shopping, a convention center, and all types of shows in the arena. There are wondrous sights to visit as well. Look at the amazing contrast as you drive to the City of Norwich and see the transportation center next to the sewer plant. See the former railroad transportation center (now home to the *Norwich Bulletin*) and the closed mill complexes (the structurally sound and the decaying). Experience the congestion of traffic as you try to make your way in search of these areas.

The challenge goes out to the builders, dreamers, scientists (especially in the medical field), and engineers, and especially the political leaders who make decisions that are long-lasting and meaningful to the overall population. They can all take lessons from our forefathers as well as other countries! (Re: *National Geographic*, 04-2019, special issue, *Cities*)

Imagine the destruction that would have resulted if we had carried a real bomb and were intent on destroying the Rose of New England. I visited the city of

Hamburg, Germany, and was surprised at the newness of everything. The efficiency of transportation systems and the politeness of the people (as well as the excellent food) are things I remember well. It is a sad thing when the grand old mills are allowed to simply fall to the ground from disrepair. Over time, they became habitats for the homeless. Ironically, several of these old mills were mysteriously set afire and some by arsonists, and some of them were turned into apartment complexes. The contrast is amazing.

Please do not get me wrong. People are trying to develop these downtrodden areas; however, they are met with superfluous rules and regulations as well as high taxes and apathy. Development is very difficult simply because of a famous Supreme Court case that occurred in 2005 Kelo v. City of New London. What happened there was, Pfizer Incorporated wanted to expand their footprint from Groton to New London. The New London Development Corporation (NLDC) invoked the unpopular use of eminent domain to secure property surrounding what would become the new Pfizer site. Thanks to a Supreme Court ruling, fifty families lost their homes. Although the NLDC had expansion plans of its own for the property surrounding Pfizer, those plans never came to fruition. Today you can travel to the shore in New London and view what is still an empty, debris-strewn field. There must be compromises in development, and if the Indians could do it, so can we.

Some suggestions to aid the people involved in development are as follows:

1. Increase the availability of facilities in Downtown Norwich, build more parking garages, and make the downtown area of Franklin Square more user-friendly.

2. Build a highway on top of a highway, like they did in Mexico City, so that travelers to the casinos would not get tied up in local congestion (especially along West Main Street). We don't need six roundabouts put into this area, which will create massive confusion, huge expenses, and even more disruption.

3. We need a fast but nimble transit system that can reach out to surrounding major areas to move people around quickly, efficiently, and economically. By doing this, local business should grow.

One possible suggestion for mass transit is to make use of an existing system that has already been bought and paid for: our school bus system. This system spoils the children by literally going door to door and operates on an average of six hours per day. Graduating students from high school on the way to college, poor families, and the elderly can move about efficiently and cheaply by better utilization of the school bus system. This issue should be resolved. As a senior citizen, if I should lose my driver's license, don't I deserve the same treatment as a child? Another small suggestion and minor improvement in efficiency is to make children walk a little bit further to catch a bus. Anyone who's ever been behind a school bus knows what I'm talking about.

Now what does all this have to do with the Norwich State Hospital shutting down? The issue of insanity still plagues our society, but progress is slowly being made as a result of newfound medications. As an example, in the past, overactive children were actually placed under lock and key at that hospital and received electroshock treatments. Now they can take a drug and attend school. Doctors, take note, insanity may be caused by a germ that spreads, and I personally feel that our politicians may be affected! Enough said on that subject!

Fear not, good reader. Soon the Mohegans will build a huge theme park for families to enjoy themselves. The new theme park will be located on the old hospital site property. The contrast is simply amazing. Maybe we can learn from the Indians as our forefathers did.

As for Wikipedia facts, they may be reduced to perhaps one or two sentences in the future, just like one bookmaker tried to reduce the Vietnam War to two sentences awhile back.

RECOMMENDED LITERATURE FOR REFERENCE

1. Images of America
2. Rockledge, Christine M. *Norwich State Hospital*. South Carolina: Arcadia Publishing, 2018.
3. *Norwich State Hospital Under Investigation bv Julianne Manein. Mav 23.2018*
4. *Damed Connecticut.* June, 2010, by Ray Bendici, Article files under Hauntings, Investigations, about Norwich State Hospital, Preston, CT
5. *Gadrean, Denise L., and MacClure, Peter Buckley. The Asvlum: Reflections of the Norwich State Mental Hospital. 2008-2010.*
6. The many articles in the Norwich Bulletin and editorials about the plight of Norwich.
7. A series of books by Ken Keeley with wonderful photos of Norwich
8. *Norwich and the Civil War by Patricia F. Stanley*

ABOUT THE AUTHOR

Wilfred Zinavage was born in Norwich and raised on a farm in Baltic. He graduated from Norwich Free Academy (NFA) in 1958 and joined the Navy. In his twenty years of service, he was one of eighteen men selected from the aviation community to become an in-flight technician on the P3C aircraft. The newly developed computerized aircraft signaled a quantum jump in antisubmarine warfare. Eventually, he reached the peak of his career while attached to Air Test and Evaluation Squadron 1 (VX-1). Here he got to work on several secret projects and left his imprint, as he says, "On every good man and woman in the United States Navy," by his submission of a simple idea of allowing gold to be placed on petty officer Chevrons. To this day, this insignia has survived. The gold represents twelve years of continuous good conduct. The Smithsonian Institution accepted the first insignia.

He retired with his family to Baltic, Connecticut. To date, he has an impressive résumé, which included a Bachelor in General Studies from Eastern Connecticut University; an actor; a TV show cohost for nearly seven years on Comcast; a selectman of Sprague; a former candidate for lieutenant governor; a biomedical technician, and the head of a test facility for power tools (AEG) (which unfortunately closed). As an armed nuclear security officer, he made the tactical response team while at United Nuclear Corporation, which also closed. The property then became the site of the Mohegan Sun casino, one of the world's largest resort casinos. He served his final years as a security officer at Foxwoods, the world's largest casino, and retired from the workforce due to health issues in 2001.

Since that time, he has authored two books, *Deployment* and *The Zinavaee Legacy*. He coauthored the *History of the Sprague Rod and Gun Club* as an active member and club historian. He is also a member of the Sprague Historical Society and a lifetime member of the Disabled American Veterans (DAV), Viet Nam Veterans of America (VVA), and Navy League and remains active with the American Legion, Post 85 in Baltic, Connecticut, and was its former senior vice commander.